PAIN

Dan Middleman

Illustrations by Kristen Hall

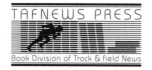

TAFNEWS PRESS

Book Division of Track & field News

First published in 1998 by Tafnews Press
Book Division of Track & Field News,
2570 El Camino Real, Suite 606,
Mountain View, CA 94040 USA.

Manufactured in the United States of America

Standard Book Number: 0-911521-52-6

Production Director: Teresa Tam

DEDICATION

To Mom
who believes in me
unconditionally

THIS IS FICTION!

While the author will admit that many of the characters and incidents that make up this book have some foothold in reality, they are all interwoven with material that came straight from the writer's demented mind.

All names of characters have been changed to protect the innocent. And the college in the book has nothing at all to do with the Florida Institute of Technology in Melbourne, Florida, near where the author's grandmother resides.

The author knows nothing about the school and wishes in no way to harm the reputation of the institution or its athletic program.

The author wishes to thank Michael Mykytok for his poems which added so much to the story. Yes, the poems read by "Mad Dog" are real verses from Mike's world famous collection.

THE REVIEWS

Ann Middleman (Mother):

"The first in a long line of great works from one of the greatest novelists in history. And I'm not just saying that because I gave birth to him."

David Middleman (Father):

"I've never been very impressed with the boy. But at least he's shown me that money spent on therapy and a journalism degree can pay dividends."

Jon Middleman (Brother):

"Buy the book, so he'll have enough money to stay in a hotel when he comes home to visit."

A friend who refused to give his name:

"I hope this doesn't mean we have to start treating him nicely."

10

The Long Ride

Richard Dubin rolled into town about 3 a.m. It had been a long ride to Arboretum, Florida from Fresh Meadows, his home town in western Long Island. Eighteen hours to be exact. It didn't help that he had moved less than a mile during two hours of D.C. traffic. In fact, traffic was so bad on that hot August day in D.C. that Richard pulled over to the side of the road, hopped out and relieved himself behind a tree; when he returned, the line of cars had not moved an inch.

To make up for the delay he pretended later that the number of the interstate was the speed limit and was rewarded for his impatience with a $175 speeding ticket outside Savannah. It was his third such violation in the past 12 months. His insurance company loved him.

The trip to and from Florida was beginning to get tedious. The first few times he had done it he didn't mind all that much. But each time the task became more taxing. He made it safely this time despite a few hallucinations on the road in Jacksonville, about an hour and a half out of Arboretum. He thought he'd be too wired to sleep when he arrived but he was out as soon as he hit the pillow at his new pad.

Devlin

He awoke at 9:45 a.m. to a typical mid-August day in Arboretum—hotter than hell with a huge dose of humidity. He got out of bed, threw on a T-shirt and shorts, jumped on his mountain bike and took off.

Richard was a fifth-year senior and a distance runner of some accomplishment at the Florida Institute of Technology. He pedaled to a meeting with FIT's head track coach Frank Devlin at 10. Richard wanted to get off on the right foot with

Devlin and show that he meant business in his last year of college eligibility. Being on time for the meeting was a good start.

Devlin was a good enough guy deep down. But he came off to most people as a wheeler-dealer type who could always sell used cars if he ever quit coaching. He didn't particularly inspire trust, especially from his athletes. Devlin—known by team members as The Devil—was the subject of constant rumors ranging from sexual harassment to paying some of his athletes. He was the most misunderstood man Richard had ever met.

Without fail, in May around the time of the Southeastern Conference outdoor track championships, the whole town would talk about how Devlin would be fired for this or that offense. But Devlin was resilient and could always be found in his office in the fall.

"I just put the key in the door and pray that it opens," Devlin would say at the beginning of each year.

Richard admired him for that resiliency. He also admired him for his kindnesses. It was Devlin, after all, who not only kept Richard on scholarship after a dismal junior season, but helped him find counseling for his problems with alcohol. Richard never forgot that and felt indebted to him. But he still had many reservations about Devlin's coaching ability, and at times he despised him and his methods.

Richard strolled confidently into Devlin's office at 10 a.m. on the nose. He had proven to Devlin last year that he was worth keeping on scholarship. He had won two SEC indoor titles, set a school record outdoors, made All-American in cross country, and was expecting a big year in his finale as a FIT Aggie.

"How's it goin', Coach?" Richard asked. Most of the athletes didn't call him "Coach." They just called him by his last name to his face and "The Devil" behind his back. But Richard showed him the respect he owed the man who'd saved his hide. Even if he did prove his worth on the track last year.

"Ricky-boy," Devlin said in his Southern drawl, thickened by the tobacco juice in his cheek. "How was your summer?"

"Good, Coach. I ran about 60 miles a week to keep fit."

"You do any racing?"

"Not since nationals."

At the nationals—the U.S.A. championships held every year—Richard got blown away in the semifinals of the 5000 meters. In an Olympic year, like the upcoming one, the Olympic Trials take the place of the national championships.

"I wanted to be well rested for my last cross country season," Richard said.

"Good," Devlin agreed.

"So, Coach, I've come to find out what my mission is for this year."

Devlin paused for a moment. Richard wasn't quite sure whether Devlin hesitated to think about what to say or to get the tobacco juice out of his mouth before he spoke.

"Your mission," he started, and then spit into a Coke can. "Your mission this year is to lead your team to a conference title in cross country and a top five finish at NCAA's."

"I can't do it alone, Coach."

"I know. But you're the leader. And if you set a good example I think you can take this team a long way."

"That's just cross country. What about the mission for track season?"

"One mission at a time, Ricky-boy. I've given you enough to chew on for right now. You concentrate on completing that mission and when that's done I'll give you your orders for the track season."

"All right. That sounds fair."

"You know, I've been thinking, Ricky. I've looked at the national rankings and I really think if you put it together this year there's a spot open for you on the Olympic team in the steeplechase."

Richard was taken aback by the suggestion. The Olympic team! But the 3000-meter steeplechase. Ouch! Nearly two miles over 28 75-lb. barriers and seven water jumps. Probably the toughest, most physically and mentally grueling event in the sport. Richard hated the steeplechase, but he also knew it was his best event.

"You really think so?" Richard asked almost in shock.

"Looking at the rankings, I think you can make it," Devlin said, giving Richard his infamous salesman's stare. But unlike most salesmen, whose stares are just kind of annoying, Devlin's stare could burn a hole right through you.

Devlin was the only person Richard had ever seen with one brown eye and one blue eye. And while the brown eye always stayed the same shade of brown, the blue eye could change intensity at a moment's notice depending on how he was feeling. This eye served as a kind of mood ring. A darker, deeper blue meant that he was in a warm, kind mood. A paler, lighter blue meant that one should stay out of his path.

Devlin, of course, knew all this, and used the blue eye with great effectiveness. A paler shade could put a loud-mouthed sprinter back in his place, while a darker shade might pick up a gorgeous blonde at the bar later that same evening.

Some believed that Devlin could control the pigment in his blue eye ("devil eye" was the term used by the track team). Richard wasn't too sure about that. He just knew that a Devlin stare could warm you up or freeze you out almost instantly. He knew because he'd seen all shades of the devil eye in his four years at FIT.

The two exchanged a few other pleasantries, asked about each other's families, and Richard left Devlin's office with a feeling of numb excitement in his body.

"It's going to be a good year," Richard mumbled to himself as he left the cool athletic offices and entered the humid August air.

The Roommates

Richard lived in a three-bedroom townhouse with three of his cross country teammates.

There was Alex Anderson, known to his friends as Gopher, mostly because he would crawl in a hole when he was sober and around women. He lost all that shyness, however, after a few beers. Alex also bore a facial resemblance to Fred Grandy—who played the character Gopher Smith on *The Love Boat*. Gopher hated Devlin. And since he was the team's sixth man—in a sport where only the first five score points—his performance and training didn't take up much space in Devlin's training log.

Gopher also hated missing a night of beer drinking and hell raising just so he could wake up early and put himself through the requisite pain it took to compete at the collegiate level. But for reasons only a distance runner —and maybe a swimmer or cyclist—could understand, he did it anyway.

An important aspect of distance running is one's pain tolerance. Gopher had none. It was predictable that when Gopher got tired, he would slow down rather than fight through the pain that comes with fatigue.

Richard worried—sometimes out loud—that if one of the team's top five were sick or injured, they'd have to rely on "Mr. Painless."

Another roomie was Jeff Rubin, a senior who was one of Richard's best friends in high school. After one year at Buffalo State University, Jeff was convinced by Richard to leave the frozen north and come to warm Arboretum. Jeff walked on the team and ran the 800 meters for two years when he decided he'd be more effective as a distance runner.

Jeff was a success, as Richard knew he would be. He was the team's fifth man, and while a very quiet guy, he was an emotional leader on the team and an example to the younger runners of how they could improve if they worked hard enough.

The third of Richard's roommates was Mike Ledbetter. Known to everyone as "Mad Dog," Ledbetter was born to be a cross country runner. A native of Maine, Mad Dog had absolutely no speed but could run like hell on hills. As a freshman he had finished 27th at the NCAA cross country championships, earning All-American honors—rare for a freshman. In the process he gained a reputation for being a tough competitor and for being as insane as he looked and acted.

Mad Dog's reputation for his extra-athletic activities far overshadowed anything he had done in spikes and uniform. Mad Dog could win a race, but would often be remembered only for the bottle of rum he drank and his howling at the moon until all hours of the morning afterward. By the end of his freshman year, Mad Dog was a cult figure in the cross country community. Mad Dog fan clubs sprouted up at other colleges, adding to the ridiculous legend.

Mad Dog was known for being a nutcase when he was in high school. This came in part because of his hair, which he kept in a crew cut on top with a tail that ran down to the middle of his back. Mad Dog also embellished his reputation when he let it be known that he prayed to Satan.

This image scared off many college coaches. But Devlin was able to look past the hair and the weirdness because of the incredible talent Ledbetter possessed. Devlin also believed at the time that a lot of Ledbetter's routine was simply an act to convince people that he was different and unique. Any doubts, though, about his marching to the beat of a different drummer came to a full stop on his recruiting trip.

When Ledbetter came to visit FIT, Devlin invited Richard, a sophomore at the time, and Johnny Reilly, a fifth-year senior on the team, to his office while Ledbetter was settling into his hotel room.

"Boys, we got a live one here," Devlin said through his chaw-packed cheeks. "I think we got him 'cause I know nobody else wants him. Take him around, show him the school. But don't go running with him. I don't need the NCAA dustin' for prints around my office again."

Devlin gave Johnny $80 and said, "Take the kid out for a nice meal and movie. Have a good time. But for chrissakes, don't get him drunk. His family is real strange and I had a tough enough time just convincing his mother to let him take a trip down here all by himself. I promised her nothing bad would happen, so please don't make me out to be a liar."

Richard found Devlin's pleading so humorous, he had to stare at the ground and concentrate on morbid thoughts to keep from breaking into laughter. Spoiled cole slaw usually did the trick. But even those images weren't strong enough to keep a slight smirk from appearing on his face. Richard looked over and could see that Johnny was going through the same ordeal.

The two left Devlin's office and speed-walked to the staircase where, safely out of earshot, they broke into laughter.

"So what you think, Johnny Boy? Is The Devil a liar?" Richard giggled.

"What, are you kiddin' me?" Johnny said in his thick New York City accent. "That redneck motherfucker is fooling himself if he thinks we ain't gonna get that Looney Tunes bastard shitfaced tonight." They laughed and high-fived their way out of the athletic department.

They picked up Ledbetter at his hotel room and brought him back to Johnny's house, affectionately referred to as the "Crackhouse." The trailer house got its name because Johnny and Steve Hargrove, a former FIT distance runner, lived in the nastiest, most drug-infested section of Arboretum. Break-ins and drug arrests occurred every week in their trailer park—which the local newspaper dubbed "Cracktown."

But despite the neighborhood crime, the Crackhouse was never approached. Even the drug dealers could see that the poor white trash who lived there had nothing worthwhile to steal; unless the street value of old worn-out running shoes suddenly rose.

When the threesome arrived at the Crackhouse, Johnny phoned in an order for pizza. Richard took Johnny's car and picked up the pizza; the delivery man refused to drive in Cracktown at night. He also picked up three cases of beer. Richard was only 19, but he looked like Johnny and used his I.D. often to buy beer and get into bars.

When Richard came back he heard Guns 'n' Roses blasting from the living room. He walked in and saw that Johnny and Ledbetter were already well oiled. Richard put the pizza and one case of beer on the floor and turned down the music so he wouldn't have to scream.

"What the hell is going on? You guys start without me?"

"We found a little cheap wine in the fridge," Johnny said. "This crazy fucker says he likes to drink Mad Dog 20/20 before he races."

"Mad Dog is the shit!" Ledbetter howled, holding up the near-empty bottle of grape wine with pride. With that, the nickname was forever engraved in stone.

After they ate pizza and drank most of the beer, Ledbetter whipped out a sheet of paper from the front pocket of his jeans.

"What's that?" Richard asked.

"I've been writing poems in my spare time," he said. "This one's called 'Hit and Run,'" and he proceeded to read:

"I lay on the road, shot by a gun
The victim of a fierce hit and run.
A dark car from nowhere, a collision so strong
Committing an act that was legally wrong.
For when I was hit, the driver pulled over
To see my half-dead body just outside Dover.
So looking down the road, to see not one man
He pulled out a shotgun with his cold lifeless hand.
From the back seat, he pulled out this weapon
On the floor in a case, which it was kept in.
And aiming quite easily, he pulled on the trigger
A hole in my chest, gradually getting bigger.
So I watched in pain, as the car sped away
Letting out a groan, for it was all I could say.
My chances looked grim, as I lay on the ground
But if I survive, I'll hunt that man down."

The first impression Richard and Johnny had of Ledbetter

was that his weird behavior was probably an act to impress people. But after the poem, they realized that this guy was borderline certifiable.

Richard's Theory

In studying the bodies of distance runners, Richard had formed the theory that they come in two sizes: those who are naturally skinny, and those who are thin only because they run. According to this theory, the naturally skinny guys would weigh about 10 lbs. more than they did if they were completely inactive, whereas the latter group would be 30 lbs. heavier or more if they were inactive.

The skinny group, of which Richard and Mad Dog were members, could eat as much as they wanted of whatever they wanted and not gain a pound. The other group, which Gopher and Jeff belonged to, had to keep an eye on their weight and what they ate even when running 90 miles a week.

Eating was one of the great perks for Richard, who could put food away like a 300-lb. offensive lineman and never worry about gaining a pound. To Richard, it was as much an issue of pride as it was nourishment. It was the one domain left in which he allowed himself to go wild. He couldn't imagine running all that way and then having to hold back when the dinner bell rang.

At the athletes' dining hall, the ladies who served the food would always have big grins on their faces when they saw Richard in line because they knew he wasn't shy about second and third helpings. Richard had a running joke with one of them, a woman, who talked about adopting him. Richard called her "Mom."

Richard's real mother had recognized his unusual appetite when he was young. She used to call him "Hollow Leg."

Richard had figured out through research on every distance runner he knew that a natural divide existed between the two groups—he called them "the skinnies" and "the heavies." If a distance runner weighed more than two pounds per inch when in racing shape, he typically had weight problems. In their best shape Richard and Mad Dog were both 5'11" and 130 lbs.— 12 lbs. under the dividing line. Gopher was 5'11" and 145, and Jeff was 5'9" and 140 —just over the line.

To the layman, they all looked like skinny distance runners. But a trained eye like Richard's could tell the difference, especially at the start of the season when the heavier guys would come to practice 15 lbs. overweight with the slightest hint of a belly. Richard and Mad Dog had less than five percent body fat and wouldn't develop a belly unless they stopped running cold turkey for a year.

While Richard and Mad Dog were the lightweights of the team, there were differences in their body shapes. Mad Dog looked unhealthily skinny, although he ate almost as much as Richard. Mad Dog was pale with tight skin that showed every muscle in his upper body. But his arms and legs were so thin that he could be mistaken, according to his teammates' gibes, for the creature that emerged from the space ship in the movie *Close Encounters of the Third Kind*—tall, white, with long stick-like appendages. Richard would tell people that Mad Dog used to be Mr. Universe before his mother threw him in a clothes dryer for a few days.

Richard was also skinny, but not extremely so. He avoided the weight room ever since he got into an altercation with an overweight football player in high school who laughed at the fact that he was bench pressing only 130 lbs. (which was 10 lbs. more than his body weight at the time). Richard uttered a sentence that ended with the word "tubby" and soon found himself rolling around on the weightroom floor with a guy who was one inch taller and 100 pounds heavier. Richard came out of the scuffle moderately unscathed, but promised himself he would not go back into a weightroom again.

While avoiding the weights, Richard worked hard on developing his pectoral and abdominal muscles by doing nearly 200 push-ups and 100 sit-ups in his room every day. Richard would complete a set of 50 push-ups and go straight to his full-length mirror to check out his slender yet defined upper body. He, like Mad Dog, had tight skin that showed every muscle in his upper body. But his body was tanner and he had chest hair. So, unlike Mad Dog, the sight of him without a shirt on was not an eye-popping experience.

He would often laugh at himself and his vanity. His chest, arms and abs were one aspect of his appearance about which he was vain and insecure.

Anthony and Marie

This was the first year Richard was living with teammates since his freshman year in the dorm. That year he lived with Anthony Williams, another FIT distance runner, who, like Richard, was now in his fifth and final year of eligibility.

Anthony was more solidly built than most distance runners. He was a very strong black man with a voice that reminded Richard of James Earl Jones. Williams, being from Fort Lauderdale, adjusted to college life a lot quicker than Richard, who came in not knowing anybody. Anthony, who had many high school friends attending FIT, had few problems adjusting and it showed on the race course.

Anthony was one of the top freshman distance runners in the country when they lived together. Richard, who was considered the better of the two coming out of high school, struggled with mononucleosis, torn stomach muscles, and severe loneliness and depression throughout that first year.

But while Richard slowly adjusted and improved over the years, Anthony had stagnated athletically since discovering Jesus Christ towards the end of his freshman year.

When Anthony found God, he lost all interest in academics, forcing him to redshirt for a year because of low grades. He had even lost, it seemed obvious to Richard, some of his will to win. One thing no one could ever question during their freshman year was Anthony's will to win and his competitive spirit. Anthony competed so hard that he vomited *during* every cross country race that year. Now in his fifth year, Anthony was not the athlete he once was. Richard wondered whether Anthony would vomit at all this year.

At the same time, the team needed him to perform well. Without the Anthony of old, the Aggies were a high-quality team. With him, they had potentially the top threesome in the country, along with Mad Dog and Richard. With him, they could make a serious run at conference and even national titles.

Richard decided not to live with Anthony after their freshman year, partly because Anthony was "born again." To Anthony's credit though, he never tried to convert Richard. He wasn't sure if it was because he was Jewish or because Anthony thought Richard's lifestyle of drinking and his interest in the opposite sex made him a heathen who was beyond saving. Nevertheless, Anthony and Richard remained friends after they stopped living together.

Though they were definitely headed in opposite directions, Richard took it upon himself to try to get Anthony focused on one more year—their last together.

For the next three years, after parting with Anthony, Richard lived with Marie Wyznewski. Marie was a tough, good looking Polish broad from the south side of Chicago. She had it all and she did it all. She was a legend at FIT. Marie walked onto the women's basketball team and became the starting point guard as a freshman. After three years she grew tired of the coach's abusive manner and quit. She joined the soccer team, where she started at fullback. She was also quarterback on FIT's national champion women's flag football team. And those were just her athletic accomplishments.

Off the field of play Marie was a drill sergeant in the Air Force ROTC. She was also a mechanical engineering major who got straight A's and managed to go out four nights a week and outdrink anyone who was with her.

There were times over the years that Marie would be out at a bar with Richard until 2 a.m., come back home, drink some more beer, and get him to the 6 a.m. bus in the nick of time to leave for a cross country meet. Richard and Marie loved each other, yet there was never a single romantic thought between the two. They were too perfect together, having too much respect and admiration for each other to ever risk ruining their friendship over romance. Marie was the sister Richard never had.

But Marie had since graduated and was now in Michigan—designing a radio that would fit inside a tank by day, and playing in a men's basketball league at night.

Richard had never lived with three other guys before and was wary about the whole situation. He had hung out at Townhouse #160 on numerous occasions when Jeff, Gopher and Mad Dog lived together the year before. It wasn't exactly a long haul to #160 either since it was in the same apartment complex that he and Marie lived in. Richard and Marie's two-bedroom apartment was in the back of the complex. The townhouse—better known as "The Clubhouse" because of the frequency of visitors—was at the front of the complex. In years past The Clubhouse members combined with Richard and Marie to throw joint parties. When the police came to one apartment to stop a party, they'd simply carry the keg—or kegs—to the other apartment and continue the festivities.

Richard didn't mind throwing parties because he knew that both he and Marie would be up bright and early, no matter how drunk they were the night before, to clean up the mess. Such was not the case at The Clubhouse, where remnants of a party could be found, sniffed, or tasted months later.

Richard was amused by how gross The Clubhouse could be with its dishes and garbage all in one pile at times. It was funny because Richard could go home to a clean kitchen. Now that this was his kitchen, the joke had lost all its humor—to Richard, anyway.

Unfortunately, Richard didn't have much of a choice in terms of places to live. Marie was gone, everyone else on the team had roommates, and Richard didn't have the money or the will to live by himself. The Clubhouse gang took him in and even let him have his own room. But Richard could tell that the state of the kitchen, not to mention every other common area in the house, would be an issue throughout the year.

"Well, at least rent will be really cheap this year," Richard told his parents over the summer.

Redecorating

With a new year came the need for new furniture. After all, when you throw parties every other week, the furniture can get quite ratty. At Tahiti Apartments—the name of the complex in which The Clubhouse was located—refurnishing one's apartment was quite easy—and free, as well.

The apartment complex had a storage facility at the back where they kept old furniture from previously furnished apartments as well as furniture left by the dumpsters that garbage collectors refused to take. If a piece of furniture was left out overnight and not taken by dumpster-diving students, Tahiti apartment maintenance workers would transport it to the storage facility in the back.

The storage room had been good to Clubhouse members and friends. Richard and Marie had furnished their entire apartment with items from storage, including the kitchen table, chairs, coffee tables, lamps, and couches. Few seemed to know about the gold mine in back and those who knew told only trusted friends. After years of taking from the "back room," everyone assumed that management didn't care. After all, there was no lock on the door. Yet nothing was taken for granted. All furnishing was still done quietly and late at night just in case they really did care and were just too apathetic to do anything about it.

The drill was simple: Richard, Gopher, Jeff, and Mad Dog would take a leisurely quarter-mile stroll to the back of the complex, walk in, turn on the light and decide what they wanted. When everyone had made their selections, the furniture, lamps, and the like, would be moved to the front of the room where it could be quickly loaded into the cars that were driven back to pick up the "order."

Every year the group went on the refurnishing run they found some surprises. Once, Richard and Marie found a huge industrial-sized microwave oven that was at least 15 years old. When they found it, they laughed at the thought of it actually working. Who would be stupid enough to throw away a working microwave? Especially one that could fit two turkeys inside.

They took it, though, just to make sure it didn't work. When they got it home they dusted it off, turned it on and the thing ran. "The Beast," as it was called, never broke down and was now taking up most of the counter space in The Clubhouse kitchen. The Beast was a great find but nothing compared to the gift the foursome was about to receive.

Richard led the way into the room and flipped the light switch. As expected, the normal array of couches, lamps, and tables were stacked up throughout the room. But standing right in front of them were two brand new refrigerators.

"Holy Shit!" Richard yelped, as the four stared in wonder at the two ivory six-foot monoliths standing before them.

"The delivery tape hasn't even been removed," Gopher said as he took out his pocket knife intending to liberate one of the two from its virgin status. Gopher cut the tape that held the freezer shut and opened the door.

"The instructions are still inside. This thing is brand spanking new. We gotta have it," Gopher said.

"Yeah, but how are we going get it out of here?" asked Jeff, the team skeptic. He had a point. Of the three cars the group had, one was a small Japanese hatchback and two were 1970s

American gas-guzzling tanks with huge trunks. None were large enough to hold a fridge, though.

The four stood silently with their heads down contemplating strategy. Then Mad Dog, normally the silent partner, said one word: "Atlas."

Will "Atlas" Heath, one of The Clubhouse's best friends throughout the years, had a pickup truck that could certainly fit one of the fridges, if not both at the same time. The four sprinted back to the house and dialed his number. He was home.

"Atlas," Richard said. Mad Dog had come up with the idea, but situations like this were best handled by Richard.

"What's up, Dick?" he said.

"We're in a bind and we need your help. We found these two brand new fridges but we can't transport them. One is yours if you give us a hand."

"I'll be over in five minutes," he said.

Atlas was a former FIT swimmer who had almost made the last Olympic team in the 200-meter butterfly. Having completed his eligibility for FIT—and having no desire to train for the next Games—he was in his first year of retirement. And in Arboretum, when world class swimmers retire, they get as far away from exercise as possible, except for the exercise required to lift beer to mouth. This in stark contrast to retired distance runners, who when done competing, generally continue to run five miles a day until they're dead or lose a leg (in which case they either get a fake leg or compete in road races in the wheelchair division).

Atlas got his nickname because his arms were so long that he seemingly "could wrap them around the world." It was the long arms that made him an outstanding butterflyer and he was often likened to Germany's Olympic Champion Michael (The Albatross) Gross, also known for his impressive wingspan.

But while the retired Atlas still had the long arms, that was all that was left of the world class swimmer he once was. He had gained 15 pounds in the first few months of his retirement and was already beginning to look a lot older than his friends who were still competing. Richard tried to get him running, but Atlas's intensity was gone.

The gang was waiting outside the front door of The Clubhouse when Atlas showed up. Jeff, Gopher and Mad Dog hopped in the truck bed while Richard took the front seat. They went to the back room, lugged both fridges into the truck, and went to Atlas's house in the "student ghetto." They would be safe there until they were sold.

The next day Richard ran by the back room while finishing up a five-mile run. There was a brand new door, a padlock, and a note that read, "Any one cot taking funiture from this storage faculty will be erested, charged with braking and entering and prossicuted to the fullest ex-tent of the law."

The Killer Week

It was August 18, a few days before classes started, and Arboretum was more chaotic than usual. Some nut was running around town killing female students in their apartments. By the time the death count reached five, the entire town was in a state of panic. Rumors spread that the death toll was really up to 57 and that the police wouldn't confirm it because they didn't want to cause a statewide alarm (which is exactly what occurred anyway).

FIT students, particularly females, began withdrawing from classes in droves and heading home under parental orders.

Richard took full advantage of the situation and waited outside the classrooms of every class he was denied in pre-registration. When enough students had withdrawn he stepped right in and signed himself up. The Arboretum murders were a terrible thing, but it didn't mean Richard had to sit at home and mourn all day.

While things were constantly nuts at The Clubhouse, they became even nuttier than ever that first week of school. Arboretum police announced that the prime suspect in the murders was Joseph Sebastian of Tahiti Apartments #161— next door to The Clubhouse. Police and media—both local and national — descended upon the small block of apartments at the front of the complex.

"Neighbor-dude Joe"—as he was called by Clubhouse members—was one of the many strange people who lived at Tahiti. Joe was an introvert. He came to a few of the parties The Clubhouse threw, but would just drink a beer or two, say little and leave. The Clubhouse members liked Joe and they made sure the cops knew that. They couldn't believe Joe was capable of such horrendous acts, although they hadn't seen him in a couple of days, nor on the nights of the murders. Absence, however, does not imply guilt. They made sure the cops knew that too.

According to the newspapers, the cops linked the murders to Joe because all five of the victims were classmates of his, whom he'd asked out but had been turned down by. Police found this out by talking to other students in the class and looking at class rosters.

The national media camped out in front of Tahiti Apartments and watched as the police drained the lake behind the apartment complex in search of a murder weapon. The gang watched in sadness as their lake quickly went dry. How many drunken skinny dipping episodes had occurred back there? How many dares to swim all the way across and avoid the alligator who supposedly occupied the waters? No gator was found when the lake was drained.

From what the gang heard, the police planned to fill the lake up only to half the level it was before and let the rain fill it the rest of the way. That was, of course, when they were done with their investigation, which would probably take weeks.

Just getting into the complex became a chore. Anyone who wanted to enter had to show a key or be accompanied by someone with a key. God forgive the resident who forgot his key. Richard forgot one day on a morning run. When he got back to Tahiti, a policeman escorted him to his house where he then had to provide identification.

"This is a real pain in the ass," he told the cop.

"You're telling me," he responded. "Try scraping the bottom of a lake looking for a knife."

The first three days of classes were suspended due to the murders. Under normal circumstances, The Clubhouse would have had some sort of get-together to celebrate a day off from school. But with police crawling around the place, a party was an impossibility. Instead, the crew spent their non-running time smoking cigars, listening to the latest release by Suicidal Tendencies, and napping with baseball bats, 2x4s, and any other weapon they could find.

Biker Phil's Party

Friday night after the first full week of school was Biker Phil's party. Richard had been looking forward to this night all summer long. It all started when Richard received a post card in New York a few weeks after he returned home from the NCAA outdoor championships. The post card had a picture of the Rolling Stones' album cover *Sticky Fingers*—one of Richard's favorite albums. The post card read:

"Dear Rick,

My name is Susan Connor and I've become kind of a fan of yours. I've seen your name in the newspaper numerous times and when I found out that you were friends with Phil Suro, I decided that I needed to get to know you. Please write me and tell me about some of your workouts. I'd really like to know what you go through mentally and physically before a race.
Sincerely,

Susan Connor.

P.S. I look forward to meeting you when you come back to Arboretum."

Richard wrote back and the two became pen pals over the summer. During the first week of school, Richard got up enough nerve to call her.

"Hi, this is Richard Dubin, may I speak with Susan Connor, please?" He was so formal, but he wanted to make sure he was talking to the right person.

"Hi," she said in a sexy yet completely natural voice. "I've been longing to hear your voice after reading your post cards."

"Same here. I've been wondering if I could see your face as well as hear your voice," he said.

"Sure. You know Phil is having a party on Friday."

"Yep."

"Were you planning on going?"

"Yep."

"Good then I'll see you there."

"Great."

"Bye," she said and hung up.

Richard about collapsed with phone in hand. No girl with that voice could be ugly. Richard had actually called Phil to inquire about her looks before responding to her post card. He didn't want to start anything he couldn't finish. Phil gave him the emphatic "O.K." and the rest—up to this point—was history.

Richard stood for five minutes with the phone in his hand and warmth in his pants just dreaming about the face and the body behind that voice.

Well, tonight was the night. Richard was not exactly a sharp dresser—he inherited that from his father. But he did the best he could. He put on what his friends referred to as the "going-out outfit."

The going-out shirt was a blue, collarless, shortsleeve Gap T-shirt with a pocket over the heart. Richard liked it because it fit him just right. In other words, it wasn't so big as to make him look like a stick figure, and it showed that he had the hint of a chest underneath. The going-out pants were a trusty old faded pair of Levis that Richard had back in high school. They were too big on his 120-pound frame back then, but had been shaped with age and fit his current 130 lb. frame perfectly— showing that he had a hint of a rear end underneath. Along with a pair of Bass soft leather boots and a black leather belt he got in a second hand store, he was ready to go.

"This is the best it's gonna get," he told himself nervously in the mirror. "If she doesn't like it, then fuck her."

Phil Suro lived with Atlas in a house across the street from the football stadium. Phil was a bicycle enthusiast who rode nearly 60 miles a day. He used to be a member of FIT's Bicycle Club—known throughout the school simply as Team Fit. But he didn't like the fact that club money was being spent on trips for inferior cyclists—namely the president of the club. In a war of politics Phil lost out and quit the club. Now he cycled mostly on his own and paid his way to races out of his own pocket— which was the way it often worked when he was with Team Fit anyway.

Because of their close proximity to the football stadium, and because of the enormous size of their backyard, home football games became very profitable for Phil and Atlas. The two could easily fit 40 cars in their backyard, plus a few in the front. At $5 per vehicle they made a tidy sum each football Saturday. A third of the money went to travel expenses for Phil's races. Another third went to the party they threw after each home game. And the other third went into a fund which would be used for future parties thrown by them, The Clubhouse gang, or the swim team.

The fact was, Phil and Atlas hated football and the football team. The only FIT sporting events they attended were the track and swim meets because their best friends were on those teams. Other than that, Phil and Atlas could care less about FIT spirit. They hadn't been to a football game in the five years they'd been in school, but Biker Phil and Atlas ruled the pre- and post-game celebration.

Richard showed up about 9 p.m., partly because he wanted to be "fashionably late," and partly because he didn't want to drink too much before he met Susan. He was actually hoping that she would be there already but he predicted no matter how late he showed up, she would show up even later. Women like that always had to make their entrance, and women who looked as good as Susan probably did were fashionable at any time they showed up.

Most of the party was outside in the vacant yard, which had been filled with cars all day. The Clubhouse gang and other close friends of Biker Phil and Atlas stayed inside where they had their own private kegs, music and places to sit. Richard was on edge with anticipation the whole night and looked at his watch every five minutes.

"Where is she?" he continued to ask himself. Not that he would recognize her if he saw her. But he somehow had a feeling that when she walked through the front door he would know it.

At 10:45 a woman walked through the door wearing tight jeans, black low-cut boots and a plain white T-shirt that fit her snugly. The jeans/shirt combo exposed the body of a hard worker. This woman was fit because she busted her ass every day. Her fitness was further evidenced by her shirt sleeves that were rolled up two notches to modestly expose two attractively cut biceps.

She was hard-core and made a beeline for Phil as soon as she walked in. Of course, thought Richard. Phil got all the women. Phil got laid more in a month than Richard had in his whole life. But Richard understood how it was.

Richard was a hard-core individual by most standards, but he also had some remnants of society still inside. Phil, on the other hand, had none. Phil was hard-core by a lunatic's standard. Phil lived the hard-core lifestyle—biking 300 miles a week, drinking beer every night, and still racking up a 3.5 GPA every semester as a physics major.

Richard ran 80 miles a week (which took a lot less time than it did for Phil to bike 300), had already been through alcohol rehab once, and maintained a steady 2.5 in journalism.

Phil's musical tastes were hard-core, as well. Jane's Addiction and Soundgarden could be heard blasting from the speakers at every Biker party. Richard preferred the more mellow sounds of James Taylor and, when he felt a little frisky, the ancient sounds of Led Zeppelin. Richard also loved a good burger once or twice a week. Phil never ate meat.

The one area where Richard could compete was in body fat percentage. Phil had 4.6% to Richard's 4.4%. But that was overshadowed by the fact that Phil weighed 190 lbs. to Richard's 130.

Despite all that, Richard wasn't jealous of Phil. He knew that Phil was a stud and was a magnet for beautiful women—like the one that had walked through the door and was now fawning all over him. Richard was not quite a magnet, but he scored enough to keep himself relatively satisfied. He would never let jealousy over women get in the way of the good friendship he had with Phil.

Richard was proud of the fact that, unlike a few of his teammates on the track team, he wouldn't change a thing just to get a piece of ass. Not the music from the 1970s. Not his conservative haircut. Not his boring clothes. Nothing. He wasn't the most popular guy in high school or college. But he had his friends, and at the age of 21 he liked who he was and what he was doing. If some girl didn't like it, then fuck her.

Richard was in conversation with Atlas, but he couldn't concentrate on anything Atlas was saying.

"What are you staring at buddy?" Atlas asked, observing that Richard's eyes were fixed on something far away from him.

"That girl's ass," Richard said bluntly. "She's solid."

"Yeah, she is."

"You think Phil's gonna hose her tonight?" Richard asked.

"No, he's been friends with her a long time. That's Hanson's ex-wife."

"No way! Well, that explains why she's so cut," Richard said. "I can't exactly imagine Hanson being married to a lard-ass."

Hanson Salinger was the most hard-core individual Richard had ever met. If Mad Dog was a cult figure for high schoolers and college freshman, Hanson was a cult figure for the seniors, grad students and anyone between the ages of 21 and 40 who appreciated the hard-core lifestyle.

Hanson Salinger was supposedly the grandson of J.D. Salinger, the author. And if the rumors about the author being a complete recluse were true, then the apple didn't fall far from the tree. As a boy Hanson was a champion skateboarder, who entered many national contests and placed respectably in most.

At the age of 21 Hanson dropped out of college, where he was an engineering major. He and his wife—her name escaped Richard—started their own chimney sweeping business. Hanson's family disowned him soon after, believing it was a dumb idea to get married at such a young age and an even dumber idea to start a chimney sweeping business in Florida.

But the business survived and the two saved enough money in two years to put a down payment on a nine-acre farm in Micanopy—about 20 miles south of Arboretum. It was after they purchased the farm that Hanson went off the proverbial deep end.

Living on the farm, Hanson developed a huge distrust for any food sold in a supermarket. Hanson had been a vegetarian for years, but when he bought the farm he decided he would never buy food again. He wouldn't eat anything that he didn't grow himself. He even brewed his own beer. Phil and Atlas called it "Hansonbrau."

Because chimney sweeping is a seasonal business, Hanson found himself with a lot of time on his hands during the spring and summer. So, his first year on the farm Hanson went out and bought himself a bicycle and started riding. . . and riding. . . and riding.

Hanson rode up to 400 miles per week that summer and, although his business forced him to cut back during the winter to 250 per week, he kept it up for two years. When he entered his first race—a 150-miler in the mountains of western North Carolina—he upset Olympic Champion Alexi Grewal. The following year, Hanson shocked the cycling world by winning the

Olympic Trials.

Even after he won, though, he was considered an outsider. He refused to socialize with the other cyclists. He refused to go to mandatory pre-Olympic training camps. And, at the Olympic village, he refused to eat with other cyclists, choosing instead to bring his own home-grown grains and vegetables.

In the race, Hanson refused to play team tactics with the rest of the U.S. team. He and a Dutchman named Erik Andersen bolted from the rest of the field (all other Team U.S.A. members were suffering from stomach ailments). Andersen beat Hanson by half a wheel to take the gold. Instead of being happy for the medal—the only U.S. men's cycling medal that year—officials and team members were angered that this outsider could embarrass the rest of the team.

Unnamed officials began spreading rumors that Hanson was on drugs. The rumors were easy to believe because of his "mysterious lifestyle, mysterious diet, and amazingly quick rise to the top." Another sign of steroids that people tried to point to was his incredible physique. Hanson was six feet tall, 185 pounds and had under 3% body fat. When he shaved down he looked more like a world class body builder than a world class cyclist. Hanson passed his Olympic drug test, but so had others who later admitted to taking drugs. The fact that he passed the test didn't remove the stain cycling officials put on his name. But those who knew him in Arboretum knew Hanson was too pure for drugs. Hanson considered his body a temple and only sacred elements straight from mother earth were allowed in.

Soon after the Games, the U.S. Cycling Federation made numerous rules about mandatory training camps being a requirement for team members, as well as rules about all athletes eating together at the camps and at the Olympics. Other athletes referred to them as the "Hanson rules." In bureaucratic terms, they told Hanson, "Don't come around here no more."

But now it was three years later and Hanson wasn't racing any more, although he still put in about 300 a week. While he did most of his riding by himself, he occasionally hopped in for a long ride with Phil. Hanson respected him for standing up to Team Fit and wished he'd done the same to certain U.S. officials.

Phil pointed Hanson's ex in the direction of Richard and Atlas. She started walking toward them. Richard stared unabashedly at every feature—her blonde, curly, shoulder-length hair, her blue eyes which he could see from a distance, her tight T-shirt. He thought if he concentrated hard enough he could see her defined abdominal muscles through the shirt. By the time Richard had panned down to her knee caps she was standing by them.

"Hi, Atlas," she said and gave him a hug.

"Hey. How're you doing?" Atlas asked.

"Good. I haven't seen you in a while."

"Yeah. Last time I saw you was about 20 pounds ago, "Atlas said, making fun of his significant weight gain over the past few months. She laughed.

The joke brought Richard out of his trance. The trance was good in a way, Richard thought. It made him less tense and he hadn't looked at his watch—which now read 11:15—in over 10 minutes. He began to doubt whether Susan would show up. And even if she did, she couldn't be as good looking as the vision standing right in front of him. He had already forgotten what her voice sounded like and was losing enthusiasm for meeting Susan every second he looked into those lucid blue eyes and studied the outlines of the tight blue jeans.

She and Atlas chatted a little longer while Richard quietly stared at her, and after a few minutes, she said, "So Atlas, have the addition of all those pounds made you forget your social graces?"

"Huh?" Atlas was confused.

"Aren't you going to introduce me to your friend?" she said and stared at Richard.

"Oh, yeah. Sorry. Richard Dubin this is Susan Connor."

Richard's eyes widened and his jaw dropped. Susan, who already knew what Richard looked like, saw this reaction and began to laugh. She put out her hand. Richard grabbed it and didn't let go. Nothing was said. They just looked into each others eyes and communicated without saying a word. The rest of the world could have burned down around them and Richard wouldn't have noticed. He was in love and he hadn't even spoken a word to her in person.

It was a beautiful, clear late August night in North Florida. Richard and Susan walked down 17th Street away from the party so they could hear themselves.

"So, who are you Richard Dubin?" Susan asked.

"Underneath it all, I'm just a Brooklyn Jew who grew up

on Long Island. What about you?"

"I'm a Louisville farm girl who grew up on the beach in Sarasota."

"So, what was it like to live with Hanson?" he asked as she immediately began to laugh.

"My, aren't we forward."

"Most Brooklyn Jews are."

"Well if you must know, I loved being married to him and living on the farm. And I still live there."

"You still live with him?" Richard said with a touch of surprise.

"Yep. We sleep in separate rooms now, but I still live out there. Although, I just got a job in town and I'm probably going to get a place in town. I can tell already that leaving the farm is going to be one of the most traumatic experiences of my life."

"You mind me asking why you got divorced?" Richard asked cautiously. He knew he might be applying the death sentence to any romantic possibilities, but he was so damned curious.

"He just became bitter and angry at everyone because of the way he got screwed during the Olympics. Instead of looking towards his friends and his wife for support, he just distanced himself from everybody. It's the way his family has done things for generations. I just couldn't take the loneliness and lack of communication anymore."

"Oh," Richard responded. Why did I have to ask such a personal question? Richard asked himself angrily.

"So now that I've answered your questions do I get to ask a few of my own?" she said cheerily.

"Shoot!" Richard said, surprised at her good mood after such a somber answer to his question, as they turned onto 2nd Avenue.

"How many miles do you run a week?"

"Right now I'm running 80." As he said this Susan closed her eyes and let out a soft sexual moan. This was definitely the girl on the phone, Richard thought, as he tried to suppress the rising energy in his pants. "But I'm going to bump it up to 90 next week and keep it there through most of the cross country season."

"When you're on a long run, how fast do you run per mile?"

"Six to 6:30 per mile, depending on how I feel."

"Oh, my God," she said and started to laugh.

Richard was embarrassed, not only because of her reactions to his answers but because his hard-on was about to rip through the seams of his best pair of jeans.

"You must have a lot of measured courses you run on, with all the mileage you do."

"I don't have any measured courses."

"Then how do you know how far you've gone each day?"

"I go by time. I can tell how fast I'm going to within five seconds per mile. So I just decide in the middle of the run how many minutes I'll run. I have courses I run if I think I want to run a certain distance. But they're not measured with anything but my clock."

"That's amazing," she said in a voice that the girls on the phone sex lines would be jealous of.

Richard wasn't telling her anything extraordinary. Every distance runner at the college level was doing about 80 miles per week at 6:00 to 6:30 pace and could tell how fast they were running. When you run that many miles per week, you're eventually going to learn pace.

But Susan didn't know any of those other runners. Richard was the first. Susan told him that she ran the same six mile course every morning at about 7:30 pace. Her fastest mile was 6:12. The idea of someone easily averaging six minutes per mile for 12 miles every day astounded her.

She wasn't blind. She knew these people existed. But she had never met one before Richard. Now she was walking and talking with one and it seemed the more they talked the more horny they became. At least it seemed that way in Richard's somewhat clouded mind.

"How old are you?" he asked.

"Does it matter how old I am?" she asked in a mildly defensive tone.

"Not at all," Richard said, trying to reassure her. "But if we're going to get to know each other, we should share some vital statistics, don't you think?" Good comeback, Richard thought.

"How old are *you*?" she asked.

"On October 19th I'll be 22. There, you see, that wasn't so bad. Now what about you."

"How old do I look?" she asked.

Questions like this were tricky with older women. Richard

took pride in being able to guess people's age, but he could tell this woman could see false flattery and bullshit when thrown her way. Therefore, the answer needed to be worded carefully.

"Well, if I didn't know you were married for a few years and then divorced for few years, I'd say you look right about 25." She smiled. The perfect start to a hard question, Richard thought. "But knowing all of that, I'm going to have to guess that you're 28." Richard knew she had been through a lot, but he had trouble believing she was any older than that. This girl still looked young enough to get carded at the local bars.

Susan smiled sheepishly and said, "On October 20th I'll be 32."

Richard's jaw dropped in amazement and his eyes opened wide. Susan laughed at his reaction.

"You're turned off, aren't you," she said, sounding disappointed.

"Not in the slightest," he said. "I don't think chronological age is the true measure of anything."

"You have to admit that it's pretty amazing," she said. "We're one day short of being exactly 10 years apart."

"Maybe it's fate," he responded.

Susan responded with another sexy moan that would have put Richard's manhood at full mast if it hadn't been there already.

It was 1:30 a.m. and Susan and Richard had been walking around the student ghetto for nearly two hours. The two stopped at Susan's car, a 1969 VW Beetle.

"So, you like to play pool?" she asked.

"Sure."

"Want to get together sometime and play? I know a cool little joint outside of town that has Schlitz on tap and Patsy Cline on the jukebox."

"I'd like that."

"Cool. Give me a call."

Richard felt awkward and stuck out his hand for a handshake, hoping to convey the message that he wasn't simply interested in getting into her pants. As they began to shake hands Richard felt that a kiss on the cheek would be more appropriate since they had spent the whole night together talking. Still, he wanted to be respectful but not appear stiff—like his dick had been all night.

Just as Richard reached over and aimed for her left cheek,

Susan moved her face slightly and the two struck lips.

Shocked by the mistake, Richard stood bent slightly, eyes closed, with his face only an inch apart from hers, and contemplated how soft her lips were. Before he could come back to reality, his lips had involuntarily gone back for second helpings. Susan reciprocated.

Richard considered himself a good kisser and every girl he'd ever kissed seemed to confirm his opinion. But when he and Susan began kissing, he realized after only a few seconds that he was playing in a new league.

The two toyed with each others lips—biting and gnawing in a soft and playful way. They used their tongues sparingly. Richard hated girls who "kissed like Pez dispensers." If he wanted a throat culture he'd go to the doctor. He had been in enough sword fights to know what he liked. And a girl who shoved her tongue down his throat lost favor quickly.

Richard was reserved with his tongue and so was Susan; they used it as an erotic delicacy rather than a weapon. Richard pinned Susan against her car, put one hand on her butt and the other around her back and began moving against her.

Susan untucked his shirt and brought her hands up and down his chest. Richard found that interesting because most *guys* went for the chest first. He didn't mind at all and brought his hands around front and caressed her stomach and breast over her shirt. As with everything else about her, they were tight and responsive to the touch.

Richard lifted her off the ground. She wrapped her legs around him as he pressed her against the car to get as much leverage as possible. They kissed hungrily and explored each other's bodies for a good half-hour before reluctantly parting and agreeing to meet again soon.

9

The First Workout

It was two weeks into the school year and the FIT cross country team had yet to do a workout. The first few weeks of the cross country season consisted of the same thing everyone had been doing over the summer—mileage—just more of it.

Richard was now up to 90 miles a week and beginning to get used to high mileage—a relatively new concept to him. But all the runs had been at a clip of six minutes per mile or slower. The team had yet to do anything at race pace. Monday, September 3rd, at the University Golf Course would be the inaugural session of pain.

Richard hated the golf course, which served as the team's home cross country course and would be the site of that season's Southeastern Conference Cross Country Championships on November 2nd. He hated the course because it was so difficult. Richard had run on some tough, hilly courses in New York. Sunken Meadow on Long Island, for instance, was home to Cardiac and Hernia Hills. At the top of Cardiac you could look across the Long Island Sound all the way to Connecticut. In New York City, there was the famed Van Cortlandt Park in the Bronx, where if the hills didn't abuse you, some crazy nut hiding in the bushes might. Richard thought he'd seen the toughest courses in America when he first came down to Arboretum, a town with relatively few hills. He didn't realize at the time what he was in for.

Looking at the layout of the golf course, one would see a course with gradual inclines and declines with a few mild hills. But no bumps, holes or divots to make one lose rhythm or twist an ankle. That's what everyone thought by looking at it. Running on it was another matter entirely.

When running a five mile race on the course, the gradual inclines and declines were never-ending and it was hard to establish any kind of rhythm on them. When racing, one quickly realized there was not a flat part to the course in which to catch one's breath. You were either working uphill or flying down-hill—no rest. On the two steepest hills—both of which you had to go up twice—there were cones set up at the top which you had to go around once you reached there. It felt like being shoved down Mount Everest immediately after you expended so much energy to reach the top.

But the worst part was the terrain. While you didn't have to worry about divots tearing up your ankles, there was a force at work that nobody but Aggie harriers knew about.

The builders of the course had put a thick layer of sand underneath the grass. The sand was put down to help drain-age and make the grass thicker and stronger. But the sand also made the ground soft—so soft a runner got no bounce back off the ground to establish the next step. To make up for the lack of energy being returned to the legs from the ground, a runner's quadricep muscles had to assume the brunt of the load. The FIT runners called it "the molasses effect." If a runner wasn't used to this, it could be a long, fatiguing day at the races, and a long week of recovery.

Richard was a rhythm runner. When his rhythm broke he always had trouble in a race. That's why he was more impres-sive on the track than in cross country. In the cross, he could never achieve a zombie state and just click off fast laps while taking left turns, as he could on the track. Cross country forced him to think about things like uneven ground, where the hills were, and where he was supposed to take that left (or right). He hated thinking during races.

The afternoon of the 3rd at 3 p.m. was a typical early Sep-tember mid-afternoon in Arboretum, Florida. It was searing hot. Out at the golf course, the team warmed up for two miles, al-though Richard thought it might be better to save energy and just start the workout because it was so hot. He was outvoted, though. Like every other team member, Richard wore as little as possible for workouts. The standard attire consisted of ny-lon running shorts and shoes—thin ankle socks and underwear were optional. In the warm-up Richard felt trapped between the sun's rays beating down on him and the steamy heat from the grass that cooked him from below.

"Five years of this shit and I still can't get used to it," Rich-ard whispered, mostly to himself.

"You never do," responded teammate Dante Ruggiero, a native of Orlando.

Days like this put Richard in a bad mood for a number of reasons. For one, he could never understand why practices this early in the year couldn't be held later in the day. At 7 p.m. there was still light but the temperature was about 10 or 15 degrees cooler. But every time he asked for a time change, Devlin answered, "It'll make a man out of you, so quit your complaining."

Richard never considered that response a legitimate scientific answer. With that thought in his head, his anger would only be compounded when Devlin would drive up to the starting line in a golf cart without a hint of sweat on his brow, and without a water jug to help the team make it through the workout. This, from a man who had been preaching since Richard's freshman year about the importance of staying hydrated in the Florida heat.

"You need to drink twice as much water as you think you need," he would say. "If I could push a peanut around the track with my nose to convince you of that, I'd do it."

Everything about this workout pissed Richard off —the time, the place, the water, the golf cart, the coach. "So it'll make a man out of me? You fat fuck!" Richard thought as he glared into Devlin's two-toned eyes.

Devlin caught Richard's icy stare and knew exactly what he was thinking. He could almost take the words out of Richard's mouth. Devlin loved it, though. Richard ran great when he was angry. He was more focused and he channeled his anger well.

"It's gonna be a tough one today boys. I hope you brought your jock straps," Devlin said.

The workout, Devlin explained, would be six times one mile with 90 seconds rest in between. The first mile would be in 5 minutes and 30 seconds with each mile getting 10 seconds faster. The last one would have to be in 4:40. It was the type of workout that if done at 6 p.m. on the track, would be a laugher. But at 3 p.m. on the sweltering golf course, a 4:40 mile after five others was downright impossible.

Richard really hated the first workout of the year. It didn't matter how much mileage he had done over the summer; he was never prepared for that first training session.

Typically, Richard would start the season competing for Top 15 honors on the team, along with the freshman walk-ons. But by the time of the season's first race, he would miraculously pull up to second or third man. And for the conference, district and national meets, he would be first, or close to it.

He was a late peaker. He'd done that every year and he would do it again this time around. But he still hated getting his ass kicked by everyone and his mother early in the season and then having his tenacity questioned by a fat man in a golf cart who had never run track in his life.

So on that hot September day, the group took off on their six-mile hell run. The workout course was a one-mile horseshoe that mercifully avoided the largest hill on the race course. The group would run back and forth on the horseshoe for the entire workout. It was monotonous, but at least it was accurately measured. Richard was anal about accuracy in time and measurement.

The horseshoe mile—like every other part of the golf course—was tricky and deceiving. It started at the top of the 10th tee with a sharp hill down of 50 yards to a quarter-mile of slight decline. A sharp left was taken around the bottom of the 10th green, over to the 8th green where the course ran a quarter-mile slightly uphill to the 8th tee. There another sharp left was taken to the fairway of the 6th hole. The 6th was flat, so a small break of sorts could be taken before a harsh 200-meter downhill, then a 400-meter uphill that went the length of the 4th fairway from tee to green. Going that way was never the problem. The guys called it "the easy way." The problem was coming back the other way.

Even though the start and finish seemed to end on relatively even ground, doing the horseshoe backwards was inevitably six seconds slower with the same amount of effort. For some reason nobody could figure out, a runner felt every slope, incline and hill when doing the loop backwards.

What would make the workout impossible today, was that the 4:40 mile would be done the hard way. Richard knew it. The team knew. Devlin planned it that way.

"Looking for blood today?" Richard asked Devlin.

"No, just effort," Devlin responded diplomatically.

"Well," said Richard, "I have a feeling you'll see a little of both."

Devlin smiled and spun off in the golf cart.

After the workout, Richard directed his aching body home. He had a date with Susan. Dinner at the Pasta Market, then some billiards and beer at the Windjammer. After that, who knows?

Susan chose all the places to eat, drink and play. She liked to control things. She liked the Pasta Market because they prepared her salad a certain way. She was a vegetarian and very picky about food and everything else, as Richard was finding out.

She liked the Windjammer because there weren't any "frat rats," as she called them. She also liked it because of their beer (Schlitz), and their music (Patsy Cline).

Richard wasn't a big fan of country music. But he liked pool, he liked cheap beer, and he liked her. Truth is, he'd have been agreeable if she suggested they play handball in a sewer.

Showered and shaved, he arrived at her apartment at the appointed time—7:30 p.m. It took another half-hour or so for her to get her act together, but he was entranced watching her ass move around the apartment as she got ready and that more than compensated for the delay. "With me," he thought. "This beautiful woman will be seen in public with me tonight. With fucking me!"

A little perfume, a little puff of weed, and they were out the door. They small-talked in his car and in the restaurant waiting area until they were seated and had ordered their food. Then her eyes got big, she reached across the table and grabbed his hands. She said in that voice that never failed to turn him on, "So, how was the workout today?"

"You want to hear the whole thing?" he asked, not sure if she just wanted the abridged version.

"I want to hear about every spike that touched ground," she said.

"Well, let's see," he said, moving into raconteur mode.

Richard took some pride in his storytelling ability. He'd always been good at organizing for effect—something he developed naturally and honed in high school and college classes in public speaking.

After setting out the workout plan, the course, the weather, the lack of water, and the smug look on Devlin's face as he sat in the golf cart, Richard described what occurred. "The first three miles weren't that tough. We all ran the prescribed times: 5:30, 5:20, 5:10. Two of them were going the easier way; so the 5:10 felt as easy as the 5:20. The 5:30 had felt like a warm-up jog. But that's where the fun stopped.

"The fourth mile coming the hard way stung. I had to work to hit five minutes. Then the 4:50 coming the easy way wasn't easy because I was still tired from the mile before. I ran that one in 4:55—five seconds off.

"I knew the 4:40 coming the hard way would be hell; and it was. I totally fell apart about halfway through and ran 5:04. After that, I fell down on my knees gasping for air. I looked up and there was Devlin and Buddy Hastings, the golf coach, having a good laugh at my expense."

"What jerks," Susan chimed in.

"No, that was O.K. That's the type of thing that gets me motivated to prove myself. They know as well as everyone else that I'll be Numero Uno by the end of the year. Even if I was Numero Nueve today." They both laughed.

"And hey, look at it this way," he said. "Last year I was the eleventh man after the first workout, so I'm really moving up." They laughed even louder. Richard thought Susan had the greatest, most pure and natural laugh in the world. She was the Real McCoy. There was not a fake bone in her body.

Johnny Reilly

On Thursday, Richard went on a morning run with Johnny Reilly. Richard, who despised running before noon, didn't mind getting up to jog with Johnny.

Johnny had been out of school for two years and had resided in the same trailer in Cracktown since he came to Arboretum. Johnny, his roommate Steve Hargrove, Richard and Anthony Williams were the only members of the Aggies Southeastern Conference Championship team of four years ago who remained in town.

Johnny had just returned from a trip across the country. According to a postcard Richard received in early August, Johnny and Hargrove ran down the Grand Canyon and then back up—naked.

On their seven-mile morning run, their first together in many months, Richard heard all about the mad escapades of Johnny and Hargrove as they traveled the highways of America. During the storytelling, Richard thought about how far Johnny, his hero, had come since they'd met.

Johnny was a professional distance runner. He didn't work. He just ran. He made very little money, mostly because he hated the road race circuit, which was the only way for a distance runner in the U.S. to make money. But his rent was low because Hargrove owned the trailer, and he never ate out. So he didn't need a lot of money.

Richard admired his Spartan lifestyle and intended to follow in his footsteps once he got out of his "collegiate commitment," as Johnny called it.

Johnny was a poor Irish kid from a working class neighborhood in Queens, New York, the son of a hard-working mother and an alcoholic, vanished father. He ran without distinction through high school until the very end of his senior year, when he popped a 4:13 mile to win the Catholic School Championships. Johnny was offered a track scholarship to St. John's University in Queens a few days after the meet—which coincidentally was held at St. John's. Johnny wasn't thrilled about staying home. But since he didn't have any money for college, and his class rank (third from last) and his SAT score (680) had scared away all other potential Division I colleges, he signed the scholarship papers two days before graduation in late June.

Two months later, Johnny went to register for classes and found out that his application had been rejected five weeks before and the St. John's track coach had been fired. Out in the cold, Johnny enrolled at Queens Community College and didn't run a step the entire fall semester.

Midway through that semester Johnny received a call from the track coach at Taft Junior College in Taft, California. The coach offered Johnny a full scholarship and an opportunity to improve himself academically and athletically so that he could possibly go on to a major Division I school. All Johnny had to do was fly himself out there and the rest would be taken care of.

Johnny flew into Bakersfield, California in early January. Taft, according to the coach was a suburb of Bakersfield, a moderately large city about three hours east of Los Angeles. The coach drove Johnny into what seemed like a barren desert with a few buildings. He stopped at one of the buildings and said, "Here's the dorm. See you tomorrow at three for practice."

As Johnny found out later, Taft was a far cry from New York. The only thing that thrived in the town were the drills that brought the oil up from underneath the desert sand. Johnny, the city kid, was now in the desert with nothing to do. But instead of crying home to Mama, Johnny did the only useful things he could do—study and run.

Johnny wasn't an academic star, but he studied hard and graduated with a 2.9 GPA from Taft. More importantly, he finished third that year at the California Junior College Championships in the 3,000-meter steeplechase and was recruited by numerous schools in California and one on the east coast. Having seen enough of the west, Johnny chose the one eastern school interested—FIT.

For Johnny, the steeplechase was a double-edged sword. The event gave him the exposure he needed to get scholarship offers. But the more he steepled, the more damage he did to his knees. By the end of his junior college career, Johnny had steepled over 20 times in two years and had developed a nasty case of tendinitis in his knees. Devlin didn't realize this until he hobbled onto campus with the scholarship papers already signed. Johnny had sat out for nearly six months with the problem and was still in no condition to run when he arrived in Arboretum.

Devlin put him on medical redshirt, which would save at least one year of eligibility and would pay for his schooling even if he couldn't run another step. Many believed his running career was over.

When Richard came to school the next fall, he was told by Hargrove, "Johnny's a great guy but I seriously doubt he'll ever run a step for the Aggies." Years later, Hargrove would enjoy repeating his thoughts about Johnny's demise in public; and would revel in his misjudgement, as Johnny went on to become the greatest distance runner ever for the Aggies.

Johnny's first season in Aggie uniform, as with most things in Johnny's life, didn't go so smoothly. With his legs rusty from not having competed in over a year, he started out the cross country season as the Aggies' seventh man after the first meet in a mud pit at the Jacksonville University Invitational

The only Aggie Johnny beat that day was Richard, who was recovering from mononucleosis and torn stomach muscles. He had suffered that injury in practice doing an abdominal exercise Devlin thought up. While Richard lay on the ground with his legs straight up in the air, Devlin took his legs and threw them from side to side as well as the ever-painful straight down.

This put undue strain on the stomach muscles, which eventually began to tear. For much of the season, Richard, only 17 at the time, took the equivalent of 30 aspirins per day to alleviate the pain. He never forgave Devlin and never fully trusted him again.

As the season went on, Johnny began to move up in the rankings, becoming a reliable third man behind the All-American Hargrove and the surprising freshman Williams. Richard, in the meantime, was a reliable nothing. But it all came together for him and the Aggies at the SEC Cross Country Championships in Nashville, Tennessee, in November.

At that meet, Hargrove and Williams ran together at the front of the pack for most of the race. Toward the end, Hargrove pulled away to win the race, while Williams faded a bit and finished third. Richard latched onto Johnny and Jon Harris, another Aggie senior, and was able to stay with them the entire race, finishing just behind Johnny and just ahead of Harris. The threesome finished 9th, 10th, and 11th. The Aggies had won their first SEC Cross Country Championship ever, upsetting heavy favorites Tennessee and Auburn.

Richard decided that day, no matter what he did for the rest of his track career, he would never have a performance that would feel as satisfying as the one he had in Nashville. That held true even four years later, after numerous SEC individual championships and a few All-American honors.

Cross country went well for Johnny, but his big breakthrough would come later that spring.

At the Penn Relays in Philadelphia in late April, Johnny would run against the best collegiate steeplers in the U.S., as well as many foreigners. Richard recalled thinking that Johnny had done well even to make it to the starting line that Saturday afternoon, because of a scary incident that happened earlier in the week.

Johnny and Hargrove were knocking back a few brews at the Windjammer on Monday night. They made good companions, because they both had a common goal: getting drunk. For Johnny, it was in the genes. He was an alcoholic from birth (inherited from his father's side). For Hargrove, it just made his insane adventures that much more challenging. Hargrove also knew that the more Johnny drank, the more likely he was to join Hargrove on some of those adventures. Hargrove would often buy rounds for Johnny, who learned at an early age never to turn down free beer.

When the two got home from the Windjammer, Johnny took off his shoes and stumbled out to the murky creek that flowed leisurely about 15 yards in back of the Crackhouse. He felt a sharp pain underneath his foot and, thinking he'd stepped on a piece of glass, hobbled inside to inspect the damage.

When Johnny came into the house he sat down on the couch that had been abused by the many parties that had been thrown over the years. Holding his foot in his hand, he watched in inebriated amazement as the bottom of his foot began to swell around a small hole located just south of the ball of his large toe. A tingly feeling began to pass through his entire body when Hargrove noticed Johnny's face beginning to swell.

Hargrove rushed Johnny to the hospital. On the way there, Johnny watched as his scrotum swelled to over twice its normal size. Johnny fainted at the sight. Hargrove carried Johnny into the emergency room where the doctors pumped him up with drugs to stop the swelling, and gave him codeine so he wouldn't wake up. The doctors did all this without the benefit of knowing how much alcohol he had in his system. Johnny was lucky to be alive the next day. But the next day he did rise from the ashes and made jokes about the scorpion sting he'd received the night before.

Richard asked him if he was going to be able to run at Penn and Johnny said he wasn't sure if he could make the trip, but as it turned out, he was as good as new the following day, the nasty bite forgotten.

He arrived Friday night at Franklin Field just in time to see Hargrove win the collegiate 10,000 meters and Richard set an Aggie freshman record in the 5000 meters.

Richard, who grew up only two hours from Philadelphia, drove home with his parents, and heard about the rest of the wild weekend in a phone conversation with Johnny that Sunday. According to Johnny, he and Hargrove went out Friday night to celebrate Hargrove's victory. The celebration occurred at the world famous "Molson Party."

The Molson Party, which was thrown at a house about a mile from Franklin Field, was not actually sponsored by the Molson Beer Company. The guy who owned the house and threw the party every year, Miller Stevenson, loved Molson beer and would buy dozens of kegs for Penn Relays week.

Stevenson was an attorney but he *lived* for the Penn Relays. His back porch was covered with pieces of the old Franklin Field track which at the time had just been resurfaced. When Richard attended the party a few years later, it took him hours to realize he was drinking beer on the very surface where he had won the Penn Relays High School 3000m championship four years before.

Stevenson was a Penn grad who had run on the track team in the late 70's. He ran Penn eight times, a number Richard would equal his senior year at FIT. But Stevenson's father, also a Penn grad, ran it five times. His grandfather, another Penn grad, ran it four times. And his great-grandfather, yet another Penn grad, ran in the very first Penn Relays back in 1895. Four generations! After hearing Stevenson's story, Richard understood why he was such a Penn Relays fanatic.

The year of the scorpion sting, Hargrove and Johnny would unknowingly be inducted into the Molson Party Hall of Fame. Richard would hear stories years later from Stevenson and others who were present, about how Hargrove was doing a naked handstand on the keg, while guzzling the beer straight from the tap—a "naked kegstand" as it was known in Arboretum. While Hargrove was inverted and sucking down beer, an inebriated Johnny came up behind him with a two-liter plastic bottle of Sprite and gave him an upside down enema.

They had a great time that night, but Johnny paid the price. He woke up the next day with the hangover from hell. At 11 a.m. he guzzled a one-liter bottle of Success—a high carbohydrate energy beverage that FIT athletes referred to as "Excess" because of its terrible taste. The drink had enough calories to last an athlete an entire day. But most of the FIT athletes thought it tasted like urine. It must have done some good for Johnny, though, because exactly four hours later he lined up for the Penn Relays 3,000 meter steeplechase and ran the race of his life.

"I felt like crap at first," Johnny told Richard over the phone that Sunday. "But I just kept hanging with Nelson [from Arkansas] and Davis [from Yale]. Next thing I know, I'm with these guys with a lap to go and I just said, 'Fuck it.' I started kicking but I didn't have a lot left and they put some ground on me on the back stretch. Then I almost tripped over the last water jump and lost some more ground on those guys.

"On the home stretch I really started going and I caught up

to Davis who looked at me and then hit the hurdle and went down. With 30 meters to go it was me and Nelson, practically neck and neck. But I lost track of where the line was. He leaned before I did and won. Then I looked up at the clock and saw 8:38.92. I couldn't believe it."

Four years later, Richard could clearly remember his feeling of total disbelief at Johnny's time, a 17-second personal best. But there was more. Johnny's time was not only one of the fastest collegiate times in the country, but it also qualified him for the Olympic Trials.

From that one race, his life was changed forever, and although he didn't make the Olympic team that year, Johnny went on to win the NCAA championship in the steeplechase the next year.

On the morning run, Johnny was going on about Hargrove. Apparently, he had entered a lecture hall at Stanford University naked with a sock over his penis—a trend he started long before the Red Hot Chili Peppers made it famous—and began singing *Age of Aquarius* at the top of his lungs on stage next to the professor, who was standing there in shock. This was not unusual for Hargrove, who used to do the same thing as a student at FIT. Hargrove would even take requests as long as the classroom was large enough and had more than one escape route. Johnny said the event made the school newspaper.

Richard and Johnny finished up their seven-miler at Westside Park, about a mile from Tahiti apartments.

"You gonna come out to practice today?" Richard said in his native New York accent that he only brought out in Arboretum when he was alone with Johnny.

"I'm not sure. You guys doin' a workout?"

"Yep. Did the first one on Monday. Six by one-mile on the golf course."

"You finish in the top 15?"

"Yeah," Richard laughed. "Ninth. I'm improving."

"All right! What do you think the workout is today?"

"I'm not sure what the Devil has planned for us today but I'm sure it's something."

"Yeah. I don't think I'm gonna hang with that. It's still the first week in September. I don't need to be rushing into anything."

"That's true," Richard admitted. "You think you'll be doing any workouts with us this fall?"

"I'm not sure. You know, Devlin's gettin' you guys ready for the SECs and NCAAs. I need to get ready for the Olympic Trials the end of June. I don't need to be bustin' balls right now. I just think we have different goals right now and I shouldn't be workin' with Devlin. I mean, if he's gonna give me the exact same workouts as you guys then he will be gettin' me ready for the college meets in May and early June. I don't want that shit. That's why I'm gettin' coached by Marty White this year. He's gonna get me ready for the big meets."

Marty White was the distance runner who started the Arboretum running boom back in the early 70's. Now a master's American record holder in the marathon, White had been one of the top five steeplechasers in the country in his heyday. Unfortunately, he was never among the top three who qualified for an Olympic team.

While it was clear that Marty still had unresolved bitterness about not making the Olympics in three tries, Richard gave him a lot of credit for channeling that disappointment in a positive manner—coaching Johnny, among others. Many of his counterparts from that era—probably the greatest in U.S. distance running history—directed their energies in more negative ways with their criticisms of U.S. distance running. Marty White was one of the few who preferred to light a candle rather than curse the darkness.

At the same time, Richard was wary about Johnny. Richard knew that Johnny was susceptible to the quick fix. He had gone astray for a short period at the start of his post-collegiate career when a mystery man named Donald told him he could make Johnny a star if he followed his workouts. Johnny followed Donald's workouts for eight weeks. He proceeded to have his first in a long line of bomb-outs at the U.S.A. Track and Field Championships.

Johnny was in a slump, but Richard knew that with the right coaching he could break out of it this year. The big question was: Was Marty White the right coach? Richard, hopefully with the help of Hargrove, would have to warn Johnny to keep his eyes open and not follow blindly.

"Do you think you'll come out for distance runs every so often? It's kind of hard imagining practice without you," Richard asked. He hated sounding like a wide-eyed, naive freshman and he hated to beg. But around his idol he couldn't help it; he admired Johnny too much. The thought of his not coming out to practice every day, as he had for that short period under Donald, disappointed Richard more than he wanted to admit. Richard felt like a six-year-old, whose parents were punishing him by not letting him play with his older brother.

"Yeah, I'll come out for occasional runs," Johnny said. But Richard already knew that with the new coach, the occasions would become fewer and fewer as the year went on. The two said good-bye and Richard ran home. Richard thought the entire day about Johnny's life since that breakthrough at Penn four years earlier—how he had changed in some ways, and how he hadn't in others.

Hargrove

Despite his four-year slump on the track scene, Johnny Reilly's story was basically one of success. His roommate's, however, was one of excess.

Steven J. Hargrove, Sr. was a leader in the meteorological field. He was an expert on tracking hurricanes and predicting their intensity and where they'd hit. Whenever a hurricane was approaching the state of Florida, some anchorwoman on the news would be interviewing Dr. Hargrove at the U.S. Meteorological Center in Coral Gables, Florida. He also dabbled seriously in the stock market, which is where he made his multimillion dollar fortune.

His son, Steven J. Hargrove, Jr., attended Coral Gables High School. Steve had been an academic goof-off in high school, but he was smart enough and did just enough work to get straight A's. He ended up graduating from high school with honors. His grades and his parents money were both good enough to get him into Yale, where his father was an alumnus of distinction.

Hargrove had run with mild success in high school. He was small and underdeveloped in high school and went unrecruited except by a few small local colleges. He'd placed third at the state cross country championships his senior year. He also ran 9:40 for two miles, good enough for sixth place at the state meet. Yet he was passed over by all major colleges because Florida was considered a weak state for distance runners, and Hargrove was physically unimpressive.

After much pleading, Hargrove convinced his father to let him attend FIT, instead of Yale. FIT had a fine engineering program as well as an outstanding track program. His father gave in eventually and started a $2 million trust fund in his son's name. Steve, Jr., would receive the money upon graduation as long as he earned an engineering degree.

Hargrove walked onto the Aggie cross country team in the fall and made an immediate impact. As an 18-year-old, Hargrove was a far different person than Richard's current friend. The freshman Hargrove didn't drink and lived to run. In high school, Hargrove ran only 40 miles per week. He bumped his mileage to 80 as soon as he hit FIT's campus. Most freshmen aren't physically able to make that kind of jump. The ones who try, end the season in exhaustion, or they get injured. But not Hargrove.

In high school, Hargrove was at a disadvantage in physical strength, but he often made up for it with a superior cardiovascular system that allowed his relatively weak muscles to get oxygen long after stronger, more developed runners were in complete oxygen debt. He also had a competitive attitude that wouldn't let him die. Although his times were generally mediocre, Hargrove was able to put aside pain and push his body further than almost everyone else.

In the summer before his first semester in college, Hargrove grew two inches and gained 10 pounds. Now at 5'9", 128 lbs., he had more muscle to go with the world-class lungs and attitude. He was a terror for the seniors that year. He came in as a nobody and finished his freshman cross country season with a third place finish at the SEC Championships. He finished the year as an All-SEC selection in all three seasons: cross country, indoor and outdoor track. He was rewarded with a full scholarship for the next four years.

Hargrove's father was not happy, though. Dr. Hargrove was upset that his son earned only a 2.9 grade point average his first year at FIT. Though that was seven-tenths above the freshman average that year, it was well short of Dad's standards. Dr. Hargrove felt running was causing his son's grades to slip. He considered the sport to be folly, unworthy of the time and energy his son was spending on it.

Dr. Hargrove threatened to take away Steve's trust fund if he didn't quit the track team and raise his GPA. Steve, who never had a solid relationship with his father, told him to take the fund to his grave because he didn't want it. Eventually his mother intervened. She somehow convinced her husband (a retired Captain in the Navy) that running 12 miles per day taught him discipline, and that earning a scholarship was a form of promotion.

Dr. Hargrove relented and reinstated the trust fund, but the damage to the father/son relationship was severe. Steve was paying his own way to school through his athlete scholarship and was no longer under Daddy's thumb. He could get whatever grades he wanted because he himself was paying for the education. All he had to do was graduate with a degree in engineering and he'd get the inheritance. Hargrove figured at the time that if he invested the money correctly, he could live off the interest and concentrate on his running full-time after he graduated.

In his sophomore year, Hargrove won the first of an unprecedented three SEC cross country titles and finished ninth at the NCAA Cross Country Championships. He also won the 10,000 meters at the SEC Championships and finished his second year with All-American honors in cross country and the 10,000m.

It was in his third year that the downfall of Steve Hargrove began. During that fall, he started the cross country season with a sharp pain in his right knee. A few weeks later his season ended in surgery; the doctors repaired ligaments damaged by all of those miles on concrete.

Hargrove was a rich man's son, but you'd never know it; he didn't own many things. He had a beat-up Ford pickup truck. He had a mountain bike. And in his room he had a light, a bed and some clothes in the closet—the bare necessities to survive. He liked to keep his life stripped down and simple. He could live without all the excess paraphernalia attached to most people. But the one thing he couldn't live without was running.

Hargrove sat out the rest of that cross country season because of the injury. In the two months in which he was unable to run, he began to frequent the bars along University Avenue. Bars which he'd never been inside of just two months earlier had all of a sudden become his regular hangouts. Hargrove had, in effect, replaced one addiction (running) with another (drinking).

When Hargrove started running again in January, he frequented the bars less, but he still made sure to take a trip to the Windjammer every couple of weeks, where he'd proceed to get smashed on a Saturday night.

Hargrove won two SEC titles between indoor and outdoor track and won his second SEC cross country title the following fall, but the right knee began to bother him again toward the end of the season. At the NCAA Cross Country Championships in November, he was considered one of the favorites going into the race, but he practically hopped the last mile of the 10K race. In that final mile, he faded from third to 15th. He had surgery on the same ligament in December and missed the indoor and outdoor track campaigns entirely.

It was during this two-season layoff in his fourth year that Hargrove made the final transition from hard-core runner to hard-core drinker. He began to see what older runners call "the light at the end of the tunnel." He now understood that his knees would not allow him to train the 130 or more miles per week he would need to run to achieve his goal of a spot on the U.S. Olympic team in the marathon. He thought he might be able handle the 80-90 miles needed to train for the Olympic 10K, but he knew he didn't have the speed required over the last half-mile to make that team. Typically, a fast 10K runner finishes his last half-mile in under 2:05. Hargrove's fastest mile was only 4:10.

Hargrove was a natural for the marathon with his superior cardiovascular strength. But lungs can only get a runner so far. In every race, legs eventually take over. And if Hargrove couldn't handle the proper amount of training for an event, he wasn't going to even try. Better not to run, he thought, than to underachieve because he could only run 70 miles a week, while his competition was running twice that amount.

When he started competing again in the fall of his fifth and final year of eligibility, he had a different attitude about his running, which was reduced to 60 miles per week in training to put less strain on the knee.

He had no further problems with his knee, but problems of another sort developed. His two injuries had affected his heart, a lot more than they'd affected his knee. Because of this, he began to tackle his drinking more seriously, while going through the motions in workouts and meets. He was still good enough, though, to easily win SEC cross country title #3, beating two

18-year-old freshmen—Terry Johnson of Tennessee and Anthony Williams of FIT. His victory helped FIT clinch their first-ever SEC team title in that sport.

He completed his senior cross country season with a fifth place finish at the NCAA championships. While most would consider an SEC championship and a fifth-place finish at NCAAs reason to celebrate, those who knew Hargrove understood that this was an underachievement caused by limited training. Hargrove at 90 miles per week—rather than the 60 he was running—would have been an NCAA champ.

Hargrove proceeded to drink his way to a sixth-place finish in the 10K at the NCAA Championships and a 10th place finish in the same event at the Olympic Trials.

As soon as his race at the Trials was over, the recent graduate and recent millionaire declared himself retired and began his life of wine, women, the stock market and an occasional run.

Sunday Run

The team was three weeks into school when Devlin handed out the workout schedule for the week at Monday's practice. Richard perused the sheet and saw the two ugliest words he knew at the bottom of the page. Next to Sunday read the words "VAN RIDE."

As the group went out for an easy seven-miler, one of the freshmen asked, "What does 'van ride' mean?"

Mad Dog and Richard looked at each other and started to laugh in a sinister fashion. "Have you ever been to hell?" Mad Dog asked.

"Don't think so," replied the freshman.

"Well, then Sunday's your first trip," he said and began to howl in laughter again.

"Devlin drops you off 20 miles outside of town," Richard said in a serious, yet caring voice. "If you don't make it back you'll probably be cut. So rest up Saturday night because the first time's the hardest."

"Did you make it back the first time?" another freshman asked.

"Don't think so," Richard replied, honestly.

"Were you cut?"

"No."

"Why not?"

"Because Devlin had too much money invested in me," Richard said, a bit embarrassed.

What he neglected to mention was the mononucleosis he'd contracted at the start of his freshman year. Both he and Johnny passed out on that first van ride session that season. They both went on to finish in the top ten at the SEC Championships that year and help FIT upset nationally ranked Tennessee and Auburn for the SEC team title.

For the FIT cross country team, Sundays were usually reserved for long runs of at least 14 miles. Most weeks Devlin left the team alone to do the run by themselves or with whomever they chose.

The Clubhouse gang and a few others usually drove to Hammock State Park, about 10 miles outside of town on Sunday afternoon. Hammock had a beautiful, shady seven-mile loop they would run twice. After running in Arboretum for a few years, one learned to find the shady loops. Because a run on a hot day was so much more difficult under the torturous Florida sun, shade often became the most important factor in deciding where to run, particularly early in the season. Hammock Park was an oasis to these distance runners. Once inside the park, Richard and others would often take off their shorts and run naked (with shoes on, of course) for a few miles.

Every once in a while, however, Devlin wanted to see what his boys were made of. So he'd call practice for 2 p.m. on Sunday and load all potential team members (usually about 20 at the start of the season) into one of the school's large vans. He'd drive northwest, past Hammock Park, to Wacahoota Road—a dirt road just beyond the county line that was exactly 20 miles from campus.

It usually took 30 minutes to get there and the only windows that opened were the front ones. Since the two front seats were taken by Devlin and Coach Luther Smith (the FIT sprint coach who enjoyed watching the macabre Sunday van ride spectacle), the runners would all be crouched into the back of the van like POWs on their way to a prison camp.

By the time the team got out, it seemed a better fate to be running than to be stuck in that cramped van with 20 smelly guys. It felt relatively cool with a nice breeze when the runners first stepped onto Wacahoota Road. But the feeling was deceiving, as many newcomers would find out.

On this particular Sunday run, Johnny and Hargrove joined the group. Johnny's coach, Marty White, had him running over 100 miles a week, so a 20-mile run was perfect for his training. Hargrove, in the meantime, had been running about four miles a day. But he was a natural talent and could run 100 miles in one run at 6:30 per mile—the usual pace for the team's long run.

Hargrove had shocked many people the year after he'd graduated when he ran 2:18 to win the Jacksonville Marathon. The only reason he entered that race at all was because some of his drinking buddies were chiding him that he was getting fat. At the time, Hargrove hadn't run more than five miles in three months. Hargrove bet his friends a keg of beer that he could finish the marathon, which was two days later, without stopping. He ended up winning $5,000, plus the keg. More than half his earnings went to pay tabs he owed to a few of his favorite bars in town.

The FIT runners took off their shirts and grabbed some water while Devlin gave an inspiring, motivational speech that no one listened to. He saw Johnny and Hargrove getting some water and decided to make conversation.

"Well, well, the post-collegiates are here today," Devlin said. "How's everything going?"

Both gave the affirmative nod that all was well. "How's Marty White's 100-mile weeks treating you," he said to Johnny. "You gonna make it through the year without blowing out your knee?"

Johnny shrugged and said, "We'll see." He was in no mood to converse with his former coach.

"And what about you, Hargrove," Devlin said. "You still puttin' back more beers than miles? I'm not gonna have to pick you up halfway through the run today, am I?"

"Don't worry about me," Hargrove said with a go-fuck-yourself smile.

Devlin and Hargrove hated each other. They'd been at odds when Hargrove started getting injured during his college career. But the relationship turned completely sour during Hargrove's senior year when Devlin accused him of exaggerating his knee problems. Such accusations were a slap in the face to a tough son-of-a-bitch like Hargrove.

Nowadays, Hargrove liked to show up at the long runs just to show Devlin that he could still run with the boys, despite, as Devlin claimed correctly, consuming more beers than miles per week.

The animosity was even greater between the two because of jealousy. Hargrove was given $2 million by his father. He didn't just sit on the money, though. Through wise investments he'd nearly doubled his money in the four years since he'd received it.

There was nothing fancy about it, either. Hargrove owned no computers or fancy phones with which to talk to New York. In the neighborhood where he lived—Cracktown—those items would be stolen and exchanged for drugs within a week of their purchase. The few times he needed the use of a computer or fax machine, he biked up to campus and used the athletic department's equipment.

Hargrove's method was straightforward. He kept up with numerous business publications and made sure either he or his financial manager in New York were in the know on every move in the stock market.

Hargrove loved to put forth the image of a lazy trailer park bum who couldn't pay his bar tab. Few knew his business side, and that was the way he preferred it.

Devlin—forever the wheeler-dealer, ramblin'-gamblin' wanna-be—was always looking for a way to earn a quick buck. On more than a few occasions, Devlin asked for a hot stock tip, but was rebuffed by Hargrove, who would make a joke then purposely change the subject.

Hargrove was everything Devlin wished he were: young, single, and rich, with knowledge and skill that could make him richer without ever having to work.

While Devlin had an oversimplified view of Hargrove's world, Hargrove didn't mind playing up the Playboy image for Devlin, just to piss him off.

Typically, Devlin wouldn't have had a problem telling a talented drunk, especially one who was potentially a bad influence on the entire team, to get lost. But Devlin hadn't given up on the idea that Hargrove might one day drop him a gem of a tip that would pay off his mortgage. Devlin also knew deep down that when Hargrove came to practice—which was a rare occurrence—he didn't come to mess around; he came to work.

The crew started out slowly at about seven minutes per mile and cautiously got faster as the run went on. The first 10 miles were spent telling jokes, stories, and occasional all-out lies. Johnny would tell a story about some escapade Hargrove got involved in two nights before. Hargrove would come back with an equally embarrassing story about Johnny. The Clubhouse crew would tell stories about each other, and about who was sleeping with the hot-looking freshman on the FIT women's cross country team.

One of the hottest topics of conversation was Richard's involvement with Hanson Salinger's ex-wife. Richard, who was usually private about his love life, told a few good stories about his experiences over the past couple of weeks. He left the really good stuff locked up, though. When (or if) it was over and done, he'd have some great stories to tell to a few close friends.

When the runners reached Hammock Park, which was the approximate ten-mile mark, all conversation stopped and a moment of silence was recognized as the runners were reminded of where they could be running—on soft trails and in the shade—if they had a coach who was more concerned with his runners' well-being than with constantly testing their manhood.

It was a cruel gesture to make them run past Hammock, and even crueler that Devlin parked the van in the lot across from the park entrance to give the runners a water break. The runners got to view the entrance to their beloved park while taking some water from the 10-gallon cooler in the back of the van.

Richard had pleaded numerous times with Devlin to take them to Hammock every Sunday.

"Do you know how much easier it is to run 20 miles at Hammock than on the asphalt?" Richard would ask.

But Devlin didn't know because he never ran a race further that the length of a football field. So he'd say something like, "If you guys ran out there, one of the new kids might get lost."

"We're gonna run the same seven-mile course three times over. The course is easy to figure out," Richard would say.

"I wanna see you guys runnin'. I can't see you in there."

"Why don't you come with us, fat man," Richard would be tempted to say. He never had the guts to say it, though.

"And how do I know some of you won't cut and make it too short?" Devlin would ask. To this statement, Richard would just stare at the ground in amazement at how this man ever became a distance coach.

"This way I know exactly how far you've gone. I know who can handle the training and who can't," he'd say. And then the ultimate Devlinism, "And besides, it'll make a man out of you."

The group laughed their way through the first ten miles in just under 70 minutes. Because of the heat and the faster pace, which moved steadily toward six minutes per mile, the second 10 miles of the van ride session were the antithesis of the first. There was little talking: two word questions, one word answers.

Devlin stopped the van on the side of the road every mile or two to make some wise-ass remark like, "Gosh, it's kinda warm out there today, boys." Then he'd spit some tobacco juice out the window and drive on. He loved to sit around with Coach Smith and spit tobacco and talk trash. Whenever Richard came to the track office he was always walking in on some trash-talking contest between Devlin and Smith. The van ride was just an extension of that.

Norma Jones—Devlin's lovable 60-year-old secretary—would say, "I'm not sure if those boys are going to give themselves lip cancer from that tobacco or from talking too much."

As the miles and the pace spiraled down, more bodies could be seen riding in the van at each mile marker. "Armadillos" were what Devlin liked to call his passengers because he'd "scrape them up off the road after they were dead."

The last five miles were merciless; running well under six minutes per mile at 4 p.m. in Florida in early September on an open road. Every part of the Sunday van ride reminded Richard of what "Cool Hand Luke" must have felt like while whacking weeds on the infamous Florida Chain Gang: the heat, the short breaks, the slave-driving, tobacco-chewing road boss.

With three miles to go there were only four runners left in the lead group: Richard, Mad Dog, Johnny, and Hargrove. Mad Dog got excited as they got closer to campus. He took the lead and dropped the pace to 5:20 per mile. His quick surge put a 10-meter gap on the other three, but they caught up to him within a minute's time.

Richard was angry and he let Mad Dog know it. He grabbed Mad Dog by the back of the shorts and said, "Don't be a moron. This is supposed to be a recovery run, not a workout. You're turning this into a race, which is exactly what Devlin wants. We're already gonna be hurtin' the next three days from this

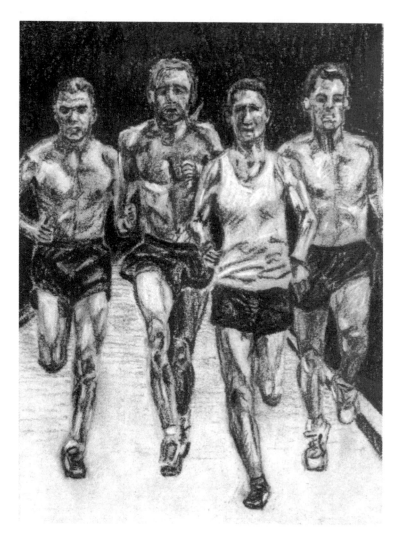

run. You go into a flying kick over the last three miles and we'll be fried for a week."

Richard let go of Mad Dog, who proceeded to take off again. Johnny and Hargrove went with him. Richard was at a cross-roads. He wanted to teach Mad Dog a lesson by kicking his ass over the last two miles. But he was too tired to go with him any longer. He slowed down and cruised in the last two miles at 6:30 pace. He ran 59 minutes for his last 10 miles. Mad Dog, Johnny and Hargrove finished over two minutes ahead of him.

After the run, only five words were spoken the rest of the day by The Clubhouse gang. They all came out of Richard's mouth. "Mad Dog, you're an asshole!"

8

Richard's Religion

On September 20th, the night before the first cross country meet of the season, Richard received a message on his answering machine from his mother.

"Hi, Richard! I'm just calling to wish you a good yuntif. Give me a call and let me know how services went."

A smile washed over his face while listening to his mother's voice. "I forgot," he said to himself. " I can't believe I forgot."

For the first time since birth, Richard did not attend Rosh Hashanah services. But the more he thought about it, the less surprised he was about forgetting the Jewish New Year—one of Judaism's sacred holidays.

One of the reasons Richard's parents liked FIT so much was the abundance of Jewish students—about 11% of the university population. The reasons for the large number of Jews were that the school drew heavily from Miami, which has a large Jewish population itself, and that the school had an outstanding reputation, which made a lot of well-to-do Jews choose FIT over Florida State, South Florida, and the other state institutions.

But Richard's religious identity started slipping away the moment he left New York. His freshman year, Yom Kippur fell on the day before a cross country meet in Boston. On Yom Kippur, a Jew fasts for 24 hours to observe the Day of Atonement. Richard felt at the time that if he couldn't attend services to atone for his sins, he could at least fast to observe the holiday. He had fasted on Yom Kippur since he was eight years old. He wouldn't feel right not observing the most important annual Jewish holiday. That feeling lasted until the next day when Richard ran terribly and blamed himself for not eating the day before. He vowed never to fast again.

Richard also never warmed to Hillel—the Jewish student organization—nor to Arboretum's Jewish community. He had grown up around Jews all his life, and most of his friends were

Jewish, including many of his teammates on his high school track team. But the reason he was friends with them was not that they were Jewish. It was that they were just like him— runners who liked to party and listen to old-time rock-n-roll. The fact that they were Jewish was more a factor of the large Jewish population in his hometown.

Sitting in The Clubhouse, deciding if he'd tell his mother the truth, Richard remembered his response to a question asked by Mary Walker, Atlas's new girlfriend.

Mary was a nice, intelligent girl, as well as sexy. Atlas was a lucky man. But Mary was also a country girl from Ocala, who had never known a Jew before, and had only seen many whom she thought were Jews on campus.

"I didn't know you were Jewish," Mary said one night to Richard. "I never would have guessed it. You don't seem Jewish."

A younger Richard would have been steamed and replied angrily, "How does a Jew seem Jewish?" And he would have gone on to other questions to belittle the person who had provoked him.

But the older Richard understood where she was coming from: a small town girl whose only exposure to Jews was on a campus dominated by Miamians.

"Well, Mary," he told her, "if you mean to say that I'm not a stereotypical Jew, you may be correct. And I can see how you'd arrive at what you thought a Jew was by looking around campus. But many of my Jewish friends back home are just like me. . . and you, too. And I guarantee you, if you met my Jewish friends, you wouldn't think that most of them are Miamians either."

Richard was more bitter than usual toward the Jewish students because of an experience Susan had at the Hillel house.

Susan, who was kicked out of Catholic school in eighth grade because she "refused to rat on a friend," said she'd always had an interest in the Jewish religion. They had only been going out a month, but Susan wanted to learn more about Judaism.

Susan planned to make Richard an "authentic" Shabbat dinner. Looking for advice, she went to the Hillel house to get some Jewish recipes for a vegetarian meal. But the students at the Hillel house didn't want to take any time to help her and rudely brushed her off.

Susan mentioned the incident to Richard while the two were having breakfast one morning. Richard, who calmly told her to ignore "those jerks," walked into the Hillel house a few hours later and gave the women in the office a piece of his mind.

"I'm canceling my membership as of today because of the way one of your staff members treated my friend," he said. He explained to the women what had transpired the day before. He then went on to say, "When you have a non-Jew come in here trying to get enlightened about our religion, it's your job to help them. There are enough people in this world who know nothing about Judaism and believe enough myths to keep them all in the dark. You people should be delighted when someone wants to learn the truth. Instead you prefer that they believe the myth."

Richard dropped his membership card on the office desk and walked out.

"Hi Mom, how are you doing? Good. . . services were fine. They were at the Student Union. . . Yeah, it was great. . . Good. Listen, I gotta get some sleep. First meet's tomorrow. . . All right, good talking to you. . . Bye."

Race Day

Richard awoke at 5:45 a.m. on Sept. 21st—two hours and 15 minutes before race time. He had set his alarm for 6:00, but on race day his body always knew when to get up -assuming he'd slept at all the night before.

Richard did his usual tossing and turning during the night and didn't fall asleep until almost 2 a.m. But four hours of sleep was plenty for him. He'd broken school records on one hour of sleep before, so four hours the night before a race was a good night's sleep for Richard.

On most mornings Richard had a tough time getting out of bed, which was the main reason he despised morning runs. But when Richard woke up this morning he was wide awake immediately—another sign that his body knew a race was coming. Richard turned on the light, although the sun was starting to rise, and moved about his bedroom with purpose. Richard was anal about a lot of things, including laying out the clothes he planned to wear the night before a race. He knew that on the morning of a race he would be nervous and not in a solid mental state, so he always had everything ready in a neat pile to give him one less thing to worry about.

He removed his underwear and donned his racing shorts. He put on the FIT tee shirt he wore before and after every race, tucking it into his briefs. He put on his racing socks and training shoes that he would warm up and cool down in. His uniform, with his race number already pinned to it, and his racing spikes were already in a small bag that he would carry when he walked the quarter-mile from his front door to the starting line at the golf course.

Richard went into the bathroom and relieved himself for the first of about six times over the next two hours. He splashed water on his face. He went into the kitchen and toasted a cinnamon raisin bagel which he topped with margarine. Then he flipped on the television and sat on the old beat-up, puked-on, blue couch, eating his bagel and drinking water while flipping the remote control to ESPN.

Richard prefered ESPN or CNN the morning of a race. It wasn't that he actually watched or listened to what was going on. The morning of a race Richard was always in a far-off land, no matter what he was staring at. He just liked CNN and ESPN because the time between wake-up and race seemed to move faster with those networks on. There were many unexplainable quirks in the pre-race mind of Richard Dubin.

After his bagel and water, Richard relieved himself again and filled his water glass once more. In the Florida heat, the winner was often the most hydrated. He went back into the living room and started stretching. This stretching was more a harmless way to release nervous energy and pass the time, rather than actually loosen muscles.

At 6:30 a.m. Jeff and Gopher came downstairs looking like Richard did on most mornings: tired and groggy. Jeff and Gopher were not as intense about race day as Richard. Gopher and Jeff looked as if they'd slept eight hours. They could sleep with the same intensity the night before the NCAA Championships as they did on any other night of the year.

Richard hated rooming with those guys on trips because he would inevitably get depressed and jealous watching them sleep the whole night, while he could only manage four or five hours, at most.

When traveling, Devlin would usually put Richard with

Mad Dog, who was still in bed. Mad Dog had no problem sleeping the night before races either, but often stayed up late at night anyway, which made Richard feel a little better. Mad Dog didn't understand Richard's craziness, but not being all there himself, he enjoyed the company of another lunatic.

Richard had a Jekyll-and-Hyde personality. While at home he connected more with the sane—Gopher and Jeff. But at a track or cross country meet he identified with the insane—Mad Dog. Most of the time, though, Richard was so immersed in his own pre-race nervousness and self-imposed hell hole, he couldn't communicate with anyone. Before most meets, Richard—a talker on most days—was a complete mute.

It was a beautiful 68 degrees at the golf course, but it would get hotter as the sun rose throughout the day. That was why Devlin always put the longer men's collegiate race before the women and high school runners. Race-time temperature for the men would probably be in the low 70's with a very high humidity that by race end would drain every ounce of water from a runner's body.

Richard always sympathized with the high school kids who had to run at 11 a.m. when it was about 85 degrees with 90 percent humidity. Then again, they only had to run 5000 meters, as opposed to the college men who had to run 8000 (about 30 meters short of five miles).

Richard walked briskly. He could think of nothing else but the task ahead. He was a machine with only one purpose— seek and destroy all competition and show no mercy along the way.

Richard made it to the meeting area behind the starting line in six minutes. He saw Devlin and nodded to acknowledge his presence. Richard hoped the nod would be enough for Devlin and the coach would leave him alone. But Devlin started walking over, clearly wanting to get an important word in, or, as was probably the case, wanting to see how nervous and intense Richard was before the race.

Richard was known among his teammates for his pre-race intensity. He was especially popular among the sprinters, who all tried to act cool and calm before a race.

"My man Dubin doesn't want to beat the other guys, he wants to beat 'em up," said Louis Martin, a sprinter. "He'll stay up all night thinkin' about hurtin' 'em."

In all his years, Devlin had never seen as intense a competitor as Richard Dubin—and Devlin had coached Olympic medalists like Martin (a bronze in the 100 meters and a gold in the 4x100 at the last Games).

One of the reasons Devlin worked so hard to recruit Richard out of high school was because of the competitive qualities, as well as the talent, he had witnessed in him. He had watched a tired and underdeveloped Richard at age 16 come from sixth place with one lap left in the New York State Championship two-mile run to win in 9:03.4, one of the top 10 times in the country that year.

Devlin always believed that if Richard could just stay up with the leaders at the NCAA meet he would probably win just on competitiveness alone. Devlin loved Richard's intensity, but he wished he could harness it so that it would lead to more consistent performances rather than the crapshoot they'd been dealing with since Richard's freshman year. Richard thought his inconsistency in college had a lot more to do with his drinking in his first three years at FIT, and his inconsistent training and mileage during all his years in Arboretum. But he couldn't deny that relaxing the night before a big race and getting 6-8 hours of sleep, rather that 2-3, would probably help in most situations.

"Ricky-boy," he said, putting his arm around him and giving him the warm salesman's stare with the devil eye. "How you feeling this morning?"

"Fine," he said. A one word response was all you'd get out of Richard before a race.

"You get some rest last night?"

"Some."

"You ready to run?"

"Yep."

Devlin tried, as he had many times before, to loosen him up before the race. But, again, he'd failed. Richard was reluctantly throwing back answers from another universe. Devlin let it go.

"All right, man, go get 'em," he said and gave him a pat on the behind and let go of him.

"And hey," he said. Richard looked up from the far-off space he was staring at. "It's a race. Have fun out there."

Richard smiled. Devlin had broken through a little, but it was only a chip in the thick wall Richard had built around himself over the past five years.

This isn't fun, Richard thought to himself. This is competition.

The entire team had shown up by 7:10, all except for Anthony, who was always late but could be counted on to show up at the starting line—maybe. He had a reputation for pulling out some close calls and sprinting to the starting line in his warmups.

Richard had started light stretching at 7:05. He recognized that almost everyone was there, so without saying a word, he rounded everyone together and the Aggie Cross Country team began the warmup for its first official meet of the year.

The team started jogging at nearly 8-minute pace and Richard felt sluggish. He wondered to himself, as he did before so many races, how would he be able to keep five-minute mile pace if he was struggling right now? He just decided, like a thousand times before, that it was one of those phenomena: when the gun went off, you became 20 pounds lighter and could run almost 40 percent faster. It was just one of those things.

The team ran a two-mile warmup that ended at the meeting place behind the starting line. When they got back Anthony was waiting for them.

"Overslept my alarm," he said and laughed a high-pitched chuckle that had annoyed Richard since their days as roommates. "But I ran here, so I already did my warmup."

Richard, the mute, shook his head at Anthony's excuse, raised his eyes to sky, and thought to himself, "Why do we have to rely on this fifth-year senior who still acts like a freshman?" Richard knew why immediately, though, and answered his own question, "Because he's so damn talented, that's why."

Anthony still lived in the dorm—the same room he and Richard shared four years ago. A run from the dorm was almost two miles, so he was caught up with the team. But it would have been nice, Richard thought, if Anthony would show some senior leadership and be there when he's supposed too.

Anthony would be worth the headache if, and only if, he ran well. Richard could take care of the leadership role, but he needed the talented flakes like Mad Dog and Anthony to run like cheetahs when needed. With those two at their best, the Aggies had the best threesome in the country. Richard knew that Mad Dog would be there. He had never had a bad race in his two years at FIT. And although the Aggies would still need solid performances from their fourth and fifth men—Jeff and Dante—the team's hopes for the conference title, unfortunately, rested almost squarely on the shoulders of the headache who slept through his alarm.

At practice, Richard led the team through the stretching routine every day. But at a meet everyone followed the routine without leadership. This was in part because most runners like to be in their own little worlds before a race and don't want to be told when to do a certain stretch and for how long. But even if they did, Richard The Mute wouldn't lead them. He figured if they didn't know how to stretch after following him for the last four weeks they were lost anyway.

He started by bending down with knees straight and reaching for his toes to stretch his hamstrings. He got down in a squat position and pressed his elbows against his inner thighs to stretch his groin and back. Then he sat down in the cool dewy grass, put the soles of his feet together and stretched his groin further. He put his legs straight out and stretched his hamstrings again.

Richard moved through his stretching as if it were an afterthought. To Richard it *was* an afterthought and it showed. When he did stretch, only at practice and meets, he did it too quickly and with poor form. He was especially hasty before a race because he was so nervous. Richard could not touch his toes without bending his knees. He had yet to have a muscular injury, but he knew if he wanted to continue running into his 50s, he'd have to start making his pre-run stretching more of a priority.

All Richard had to do was look at Johnny's coach, Marty White, to know what he would look like as an older man if he didn't start doing flexibility exercises. Watching Marty run was painful. Once a great distance runner, Marty's back was so stiff now, he could only hobble five miles about three times a week. Yet the man still didn't stretch.

Richard took off his training shoes and put on his racing spikes. He loved putting on the spikes. They were so light he felt like he was running barefoot but without the pain to the soles of his feet. Maybe it's the spikes, he thought, still trying to solve that mystery of why you lose the imaginary 20 pounds between the warmup and the race.

He got up and half-assed a few 70-meter strides to simulate the nervous sprint that inevitably occurs when the gun goes off—a ritual he usually didn't participate in.

Why does that happen? he wondered while walking back to the starting line after his first stride. Why do most people break into a sprint at the start of five a mile race? And why is it that the slower runners tend to go out the fastest? Certainly, they know they can't win. Maybe they're just looking for the 15 minutes of fame that Andy Warhol promised them.

Cross country is so odd that way. A look at the positioning in the first quarter-mile of a cross country race is often the inverse of the positioning at the finish. The slow guys sprinting in front, with the fast guys relaxing in back. Richard rarely sprinted at the start of any race over a mile. (Anything under a mile *was* a sprint to Richard.) He always figured the more energy he used at the start, the less he would have left for the end.

One way his pre-race nerves helped him in a race was that they actually weighed him down at the start. When he was really nervous, his body was not prepared to make a mad dash from the gun. The nerves had a numbing effect on him, which didn't wear off until about a half-mile into the race. Richard often found himself well back at that point but his body was a lot fresher than those in front of him, most of whom he would pass less than a mile later.

No one was more of a master at the "slow and steady wins the race" strategy than Richard's chief competitor in the SEC, Terry Johnson of Tennessee. At big meets Richard would usually catch up with the lead pack by the mile mark. At two miles, Johnson would stroll up casually, say something like, "Time to go boys," and blow everyone off the course.

Johnson was a tough son-of-a-bitch, a worthy adversary. Richard liked to race him because he always ran well against Johnson, even if he lost—which was most of the time on the track and all of the time in cross country.

Richard was walking back to the starting line when a tense Devlin called the team together. Everyone wearing an FIT uniform came together and put their hand into the middle of the tight circle they had created. The circle was the most intense time for Richard. Devlin would say something meant to psych up the team (if anyone was actually listening). After the pep talk Devlin would say, "On three. One, two, three," and the team would shout, "F-I-T, FIGHT!" Devlin had come up with that during Richard's freshman year. Richard liked the chant, even though he never got caught up in Devlin's pre-race pep talks, which sounded like they were more suited for a football team.

In the circle, most guys focused their eyes on the pile of hands in the middle, not wanting to look at anyone else. Richard liked to occasionally look around at his teammates faces. Even the coolest guys under pressure were vulnerable in the circle.

One image that was burned indelibly in Richard's mind was of Hargrove, Johnny, and Jon Harris in the circle before the SEC Cross Country Championships four years ago. It was their senior year and Devlin gave a pep talk about "doing it for the seniors." It was one pep talk everyone listened to. During that speech, Richard sneaked a peek at the three seniors. The three, who never seemed to be bothered by anything before or after a race no matter what the outcome, had tears in their eyes. It was then that Richard, 17 at the time, realized the seriousness of the matter. After seeing that, Richard would have thrown himself in front of a speeding truck for those guys.

"FIGHT!" they shouted, and the team lined up at the starting line at their assigned spot.

"There will be one command," said John Jenkins, the elderly official, over the megaphone. The old man had given this very speech about 10,000 times in his 40-something years of officiating. "I'll say 'SET' and then I'll shoot the gun. If someone falls within the first 100 meters, I'll shoot the gun again and we'll start over. Good luck."

"Runners set."

Richard toed the line with his left foot, putting his right foot in back. He bent his knees slightly, held his arms out so they'd be ready to move, and put his head down to listen for the sound of the gun.

"BANG!"

Richard pushed off with his back foot and started out on the journey. He got out surprisingly fast and was in the top three within the first 200 meters. He attributed that to the lack of strong competition at this meet. Richard then settled in behind Mad Dog and let him lead the way.

Richard often tried to become hypnotized by the person in front of him to help himself forget about the pain. The trick often worked in the longer races on the track, but it never seemed to work in cross country, especially on the home course. Mad Dog, Richard, Anthony, and a host of other stragglers floated through the first mile marker in 5:00. Richard felt relaxed, but that would soon change.

Just after the mile marker the group began their ascent up the nasty hill at the end of the horseshoe. The group went up the hill, around the cones which surrounded the putting green, and back down the steep hill. Richard began huffing and puffing and could feel the rising sun deliver its heat. The course was relentless from here to the finish: either up or down with very few breaks.

The group reached two miles in 10:10. Richard cursed in frustration because he worked so much harder on the second mile than the first and ran 10 seconds slower. He'd always had a suspicion that the course's two-mile mark was long.

The lead group was beginning to dwindle at two miles. As they rounded the lake, Mad Dog opened a three-second lead on Richard, Anthony, and one guy from Florida State. Richard was getting more frustrated as his legs fell into that weakened state that only occurred on his home course—a course he hated intensely. He put his head down and took his frustrations out on the next hill, making up the gap on Mad Dog, and opening one up on Anthony and the FSU runner.

Richard was great at running uphill because he had short strides and good knee lift. But because of that form he was a terrible downhill runner. When the two leaders rounded the cones at the top of that hill and began to descend, Mad Dog opened the lead back up and the two he'd left just a minute ago were right with Richard again. He was back where he started, with a lot less energy than he had before.

The group reached the three-mile mark (located just past the starting line). It was there that most of the spectators stood to watch the race. Richard saw Susan and Phil, but couldn't process any thoughts about them because he was too tired to think about anything but the lousy feeling one gets from running on this course. They shouted something to him, in words he couldn't understand. Undoubtely, words of encouragement, he thought.

Past three miles, Richard concentrated on keeping his form, not falling apart, and beating Anthony and the FSU runner. Mad Dog was going to beat him, he'd already accepted that. He could handle losing the first race or two to Mad Dog. He didn't honestly expect to beat him coming into the race. But losing to Anthony would be too much, especially after he'd slept through his alarm.

By the time Richard reached the four-mile mark (which was just ahead of the one-mile mark on the backside of the horseshoe) Mad Dog had a 15-second lead on him, and Anthony and the FSU guy were still hanging on. Richard decided to put in a surge to see what he and the other two were made of.

Up the hill, then down the hill, then a cut over to the other big hill. Richard put his head down and charged, gaining huge chunks of ground on the ups and losing a little of it on the downs. But the strategy had worked. With a half-mile to go he'd opened a 10-second lead on the two behind him and closed the gap on Mad Dog to a mere 10 seconds. He was pretty well spent, but he had enough to hold on for second.

Richard ambled into the finish chute in 25:14, his fastest time ever on the home course. He finished 12 seconds behind Mad Dog and six ahead of Anthony, who had to sprint the last 200 meters to beat the FSU runner by two seconds.

Richard needed help through the chute and to a massage table where they sat him down and threw a cold, wet towel over his head. Richard felt sleepy but the trainers wouldn't leave him alone. They forced him to drink water, and asked him questions like, "Are you all right?" and "Do you need more water?"

Richard was too tired to think, let alone answer questions about his physical well-being. He just ignored the questions, went on drinking water, and enjoyed the coolness of the towel. After about 10 minutes, when Richard recovered his wits, he went over to the rest of the team. Most of the guys looked about as tired as Richard felt. They all had a drained look in their eyes that said, "I've just been to hell and back and now all I want to do is find my bed and go to sleep."

Only Mad Dog looked unfazed. He looked the same as he did before the race, only a little wetter. Richard looked at Mad Dog, who said, "It's fucking hot out here."

Richard cracked a smile— his first of the day. He was beginning to snap out of the race trance and turn back into the Richard Dubin he was six-and-a-half days out of the week.

Devlin gathered the team together and told them he was pleased with the effort they produced. Even Richard, a pessimist by nature, had to admit the team looked strong. The fifth man, Jeff, finished in 26:30. They would need to improve their times to win the conference meet, but the general opinion was that it was a successful first outing for the Aggies.

Richard walked back with his three roommates to The Clubhouse. They showered, changed, and walked across the street to Charlie's Pizza Palace for the all-you-could-stuff-your-face-without-puking buffet. It was only 11 a.m. There were many days when Richard would just be venturing out of bed at 11 a.m. But the crew had already been through a full day and now it was "Miller Time," as Jeff would say. Jeff was always available with a line from the late 70s/early 80s that was incredibly cheesy, yet completely apropos.

Richard loved this time: after a race, going with your teammates to a buffet and gorging yourself with food and laughter, then returning to the homestead and taking a team nap.

It reminded Richard of the knights of medieval times. Go out. Fight a battle. Come back to the castle for a magnificent feast. Lie down to rest for a while. Then party all night. It was this camaraderie among athletes that Richard enjoyed most about athletics. He loved the battle, the competition. And he especially loved to run fast—which is why he liked the track (where your time is everything) better than cross country (where different courses mean very different times). But it was those times after the battle that he would remember most fondly.

After the buffet, Richard napped for nearly four hours. He awoke at 4 p.m. and called Susan.

"Hi," she said in The Voice. "You were awesome today."

"Thanks," Richard said humbly.

"Did you hear what I said to you at the three-mile mark?"

"No, I couldn't hear anything," he said. "I was in a world of hurt by that point."

"I said, 'You've got The Power.' And right after that you picked it up and dusted those two guys."

"I suppose they were just more hurting than I was."

"Listen, I was just getting up from a nap," she said. "Why don't you come over, hop in bed and tell me about everything that went through your bad-ass mind today."

"Well, I'm not sure I remember all that much. My mind typically goes blank before, during and after a race. But that bed part sounds like fun."

She laughed The Laugh.

"I'll be over directly," he said.

He hung up the phone, grabbed his car keys and was out

the door.

Richard drove across town and was upstairs in a flash. Stepping out of his flipflops and peeling off his T-shirt and shorts, he tunneled under the covers on the far side of the bed and slithered across the queen-size futon to her warm and waiting form.

"Why don't you take these things off," she said and snapped the elastic band of his Jockey briefs, just in case he didn't know what she was referring to. Richard complied quickly and slid beneath the lovely body and the two were fully entwined.

"So, tell me everything you were thinking durng the race," she said.

Richard, who was thinking about how warm her thighs felt around his waist, had more urgent matters on his mind than the race.

"I was thinking that I wanted to get the race over quickly so I could come over here and lick every square inch of your body like a postage stamp."

"The moan" emanated from Susan, and Richard flipped her over and the tip of his tongue began its exquisite journey.

7

Dick Stomp

On the cool-down after the Florida State Invitational, Richard realized the season was flying by. The meet was the team's third of year. They had yet to lose, although they had a close one-point victory over Virginia at the UVA Invitational two weeks earlier.

The reason for the close victory was Anthony, who faded from fourth to 14th place in the last mile. But with Mad Dog finishing first, Richard nine seconds back in second, and Dante and Jeff finishing right behind Anthony, the Aggies were able to pull out the victory.

At the FSU meet, Mad Dog won again, but was only six seconds ahead of Richard, confirming to Richard that he was headed in the right direction. Within the next two meets—the FIT Invite or the SEC Championships—he knew he would get the better of Mad Dog.

Richard liked the FSU meet. The course was easy and fast, and the meet was traditionally held on the Friday of FIT's homecoming, which happened to be the weekend of Richard's birthday. His birthday was always the occasion for the wildest party of the fall semester. This year, Friday's party would fall exactly on his birthday.

Richard's birthday party, better known as "Dick Stomp," had become a tradition in Arboretum. The party, which usually started around 11 p.m., was named after the Aggie Stomp: the huge pep rally held the eve of the homecoming game at which the 70,000-seat football stadium is packed with students, alumni and other Aggie fanatics listening to comedians and watching fraternities and sororities do more or less comical skits that make fun of everyone from the President of the United States to the President of Florida State University, FIT's hated rival.

Dick Stomp started Richard's second year on campus when he arrived back at his apartment after Aggie Stomp. He walked right into a surprise party for his 19th birthday Marie had thrown for him. The inaugural Dick Stomp turned into a throw-your-beer-on-your-date kegfest. The next year the party was expanded to Biker Phil and Atlas's house. At 3 a.m., a girl who was in a journalism class with Richard walked into the living room and found everyone present dancing in a clothes-optional format, with very few exercising the option.

The girl, who also happened to be a staff writer for the school paper "The Agrarian," wrote a front page article about the party, labeling it a "60's-style orgy." When people read the word "orgy" the curiosity level escalated. The next year more than 500 showed up. Richard figured that they'd gone through 19 kegs that night. But most people were disappointed to learn it was mostly a bunch of naked guys running around and doing upside-down keg stands, rather than a true orgy.

On the two-hour van ride home from the FSU meet, Richard, Gopher, Jeff, and Mad Dog figured that ten kegs would probably do it for this year's Dick Stomp. They would collect enough money for four kegs to start the party off and collect money throughout the night for any additional needs.

When the van dropped the four Clubhouse residents off at Tahiti Apartments, they walked in the door, threw down their spikebags, grabbed their wallets, and drove across the street to the supermarket in Richard's car.

Once in the store, they worked as a team. Richard and Jeff, the two members of legal age, went to the front counter to check on keg prices. The priority in this situation was clear: quantity over quality. The justification was that after three or four beers, the cheapest pisswater out of Milwaukee tasted like the most expensive foreign brew—as long as it was cold. So why pay for quality when your taste buds can't tell the difference anyway?

Gopher and Mad Dog went around buying the other essentials: cups, chips, dips, and anything else they could justify spending money on as a party necessity. After about 15 minutes, Gopher and Mad Dog made it through the checkout counter and walked up to Richard and Jeff, who were still at the counter waiting for their four kegs of Milwaukee's cheapest. As they got closer, Richard could see childish smirks on his younger roommates' faces.

"What did you get?" Richard asked warily.

Mad Dog pulled a finger painting kit from a paper bag. "Dude," he said. "Let's paint the walls tonight." Richard looked at Jeff, whose eyes were glowing with the possibilities. He could tell it was going to be one of those nights.

"Don't you think we should put up some paper to protect the walls?" Richard asked.

"Why bother," Mad Dog reasoned. "We're gonna have to paint the walls at the end of the year anyway."

"What about the carpet?" Richard asked.

"It's watercolor. We can wash it out," Mad Dog said. Richard thought for a moment and couldn't believe he was consulting Mad Dog on this matter. He couldn't believe Mad Dog was putting together coherent sentences about a subject within the realm of reality. Usually, logical connection came to Mad Dog only when he talked about Greek and Roman mythology or his hatred for Devlin. Richard couldn't believe that Mad Dog's answers were actually making sense.

Finally, Richard said, "Let's do it."

Jeff and Gopher gave an excited "Woohoo," threw up their hands and high-fived each other.

"It's going to be an interesting evening," Richard said to himself.

Richard and Jeff drove back to the apartment. Richard drove slowly with his emergency lights flashing because he had four kegs rolling around in back. Mad Dog and Gopher walked the 200 meters back because there wasn't enough room for them and the kegs in the car. Plus, they got tired of waiting around for the kegs and wanted to go home and crank up some Guns N' Roses to release some of their pre-party excitement.

Richard enjoyed moments alone with Jeff. They'd known each other since the first grade when Jeff moved to Fresh Meadows from Brooklyn. Because their parents were so close, they did everything together—even when they didn't get along for a few years in the late elementary school and early junior high years. But since high school, Richard and Jeff, along with Jason, another lifelong friend from Fresh Meadows, were best friends.

Richard, Jeff and Jason were more like brothers because none of them had siblings they could relate to. Jeff had a sister who was six years older. Jason had a brother who was two years younger, but they hated each other. Richard's brother, Evan, was nearly eight years younger. Richard hadn't seen his brother for more than a few weeks at a time since he went away to college. Evan was 10 at the time. Now he was 14 and competing on the varsity wrestling team as an eighth grader.

So much had changed in Evan's life since Richard moved away that he felt like he didn't even know his brother. He followed Evan's growth as a person over the past four years through the phone line. He thought his relationship with Evan was more characteristic of cousins than of brothers, but there was no way to change it. He certainly wasn't going to move back home anytime soon. Not only would he be miserable at his parents' home, but that move would damage his relationship with Evan, who had gotten used to being an only child and having the entire upstairs of the house to himself.

A while ago, Richard had decided that it was the age difference that made the brothers Dubin so distant. If he'd stayed at home all these years he'd know his brother a lot better. They'd also probably hate each other by now. He figured they were better off being far away from each other.

The distance between Evan and him had brought Richard even closer to Jeff and Jason since they graduated from high school, even though Jason attended college in upstate New York. Richard didn't communicate how he felt to a lot of people, so he needed a brotherly figure or two to confide in. Jeff and Jason filled that role.

"Are you going to Aggie Stomp tonight?" Jeff asked Richard on the short but slow ride home from the supermarket.

"I doubt it. I've gone four years in a row. The act is growing old. What about you?"

"I'll probably go up there and scalp a ticket. It's my last one; I might as well go. Hey, is Susan going to come to Dick Stomp?"

"Uh, uh," Richard grimaced.

"Uh, oh. Maybe I shouldn't have asked," Jeff said.

"She said she doesn't like 'beer-guzzling pukefests.'" Richard used his first two fingers on each hand to emphasize that he was quoting her directly.

"Instead, she's going to a party being thrown by one of her artsy, granola-head, hairy-legged, new wave, wine-and-cheese girlfriends—of which she has many," Richard said bitterly. "It's a mostly girls thing with a few gay guys thrown in for good measure." Richard was getting more pissed as he talked.

"You know what really gets me Jeff? It's not that she's going to that other party. I mean, I don't need her attendance to legitimize my party. And I'm definitely not the jealous boyfriend type. You know that. It's that she knows that it would make my night if she showed up, yet she won't show for that very reason. I also don't like the way she turns her nose up at our party, when she's the one who'll wake up with the bigger hangover in the morning.

"I'm beginning to see some bad patterns developing in this relationship," Richard said. "You know, we have yet to do one activity that I suggest. I mean, I enjoy doing the things that she suggests even if I don't like the activity all that much. I do it just because I want to be around her. But it seems that any time I suggest something, even if it's an activity that we've done before—which means she suggested it in the first place—she's automatically not in the mood. She has to suggest the idea every time in order for her to agree to do it.

"I noticed this trend early on, but I was so hot for her I didn't give a shit. Now I really want to get this relationship on equal footing. And every time I try to take a step in that direction an argument ensues. We've had a lot of arguments lately, particularly over that issue.

"Sometimes I think she doesn't even want to date me," he continued. "But she's so inconsistent with her affections it's hard to tell. Sometimes I come over and she's all over me. Other times I'm invisible. It's that way when we go out too. Some nights she'll be grabbing my dick under the table. Other nights she'll see friends when we walk in and I won't see her for the next couple of hours.

"She talks about our future sometimes. She says we'll be 'friends for life' and we'll always keep in touch. I laugh at her when she says it. I am just afraid that some day she's gonna call my bluff. And then I don't know what I'll do. I've never felt this way about anyone before. Right now I can't see living without her. But I'm having trouble seeing this relationship last forever.

"You know, during one of our arguments, I told her that while she controls the relationship now, I would control the way it ends. You wouldn't believe how that kills her. Shit, she's still friends with all her old boyfriends and her ex. She doesn't know what it's like to lose touch with someone she's been intimate with. That fear of total rejection might be the only reason she's still allowing me the privilege of fucking her.

"But I'll tell you what, Jeff. No matter how it ends, even

under the best conditions, it's gonna be painful. Especially for me."

Richard and Jeff had been parked in front of the apartment and sitting in the car for almost 10 minutes. Richard looked over at Jeff and could see he was uncomfortable. He thought that Jeff was probably sorry he'd asked about Susan. Richard's anger had passed and now he talked in a somber tone.

"You know, she warned me from the start not to get too close to her. She said she might just decide to take off some day and I shouldn't get too attached. Unfortunately, I passed 'too attached' about two weeks into the relationship. This could end up ugly."

The two sat in the car in complete silence for over a minute while the weight of Richard's last statement settled in on both of them. Finally, Jeff spoke.

"Come on, let's get the kegs. We've got a pukefest to throw tonight."

The two laughed, got out of the car and lugged in the kegs one by one.

By 7 everything was ready. All the furniture worth saving was thrown in Richard's room. The torn-up, puked-on couch was kept in the living room, assuring it would get even more torn up and puked on. Richard wanted to put that couch in one of the three upstairs bedrooms to save it from any further damage. He was outvoted, though. They didn't feel it was worth the effort because it was so heavy to move.

They hid all valuables in the little nooks and crannies of their rooms, and left as little as possible in the refrigerator so the drunken zombies who get hungry after midnight wouldn't have a feast at Clubhouse expense. The four Clubhouse members sat on the puke couch which was conveniently situated next to the one keg that had been tapped. They sipped beer, watched the sunset, and talked about how cold it was supposed to get.

Jeff, who decided he was too lazy to bike up to the stadium and scalp an Aggie Stomp ticket, said it was supposed to dip below 40 degrees that night. "Good," Richard said, "the beer will stay cold." He also knew that with the hundreds of people who would be packed into their apartment like sardines in a can within a matter of hours, a cool breeze would feel refreshing.

Richard loved it when a cold front came through Arboretum. It gave him just a little taste of home, a little break from the almost unending chain of hot, humid days that dominated the north Florida weather map. He also loved it when the Miamians, who comprised half the student population at FIT, would show up to class in winter jackets when the mercury dipped below 60 degrees.

Richard thought Floridians, particularly those from the southern part of the state, were the wimps of world. He never heard so many people gripe about the weather until he came to Florida. He suspected that many of the newcomers to Florida—of which there were many—came because they were tired of the cold weather in New York. Richard thought that using weather as a primary reason for moving was weak. And although he had relatives in Miami with whom he was close, his opinion was that students at FIT from Miami were generally feeble.

Of course, Richard had to admit that even he could be susceptible to cold-weather willies. When he left Long Island after high school, he thought he could live without ever seeing cold weather again. He remembered his two recruiting trips in high school. The first was to FIT and the second to Penn State. The temperature when he visited Arboretum in November was 75 degrees and mildly humid. When he visited Penn State in January it was 18 degrees and snowing. No contest. He was Florida bound.

But after four years of constant heat, with only occasional breaks for rain and slightly chilly weather, he wanted a little cold. He liked the idea of feeling the cold against his face while the rest of his bundled-up body was toasty warm. He believed that you couldn't truly appreciate warm weather unless you had to withstand a little cold weather.

"So tonight it's supposed to be cold," he said to the keg sitting next to him. "Good, maybe I'll get to break out one of my sweaters."

The trickle of people into The Clubhouse was slow at first. At 10:30 p.m. only about 20 people were there. Aggie Stomp had been over for a half-hour and not many people had shown up. Richard was beginning to fear the worst; nobody was coming. The party will be a bust and we'll have three full kegs left, he thought.

While paranoid thoughts ran through Richard's head, he knew deep down it would be a good party. He'd never thrown a bad one in his life—high school or college. "If you throw it, they will come," was the slogan. Richard knew they were just taking their time getting there.

An hour later the place was packed. Richard couldn't move through his own living room, and settled on a spot outside on the porch. Jeff punched some holes in a metal garbage can, threw some wood in, and started a fire outside. People gathered around the fire and talked and drank.

Richard was trying to pace himself so he wouldn't wake up in the morning wishing he were dead. But he was getting caught up in the festivities and had already downed five beers from his 16-ounce glass mug before midnight. He knew then that he was in trouble unless he put on the brakes soon.

Everyone was there that Richard wanted to see: Atlas and Mary, Biker Phil, Dante, all the swimmers and most of the track guys. Marie had even driven down from Michigan for the party. She entertained herself, as did most of the guests, by painting the walls. Johnny and Hargrove were in fine form. Both were loaded and beginning to entertain thoughts of raising hell with Atlas and Phil as they stood by the fire.

Richard even had some surprise visitors. Anthony Williams, Mr. Sobriety, showed up for a little while, hung out, left his writing on the wall and departed after about a half-hour.

Richard knew it was a good party when Hanson Salinger showed up on his bike just after midnight. Richard offered Hanson some finger paint, but he declined, saying he didn't feel up to vandalism on that particular night. Richard stood against the porch door and stared at Hanson, who was over by the fire drinking with Phil and Atlas. He had biked the 20 miles from his house to Tahiti Apartments and would bike back after he downed a few of his homemade brews with his friends.

Richard admired everything about Hanson. He was clad in overalls, a sweatshirt, and hi-top Chuck Taylors with wool socks. The bottom of his overalls were tucked into his wool socks to maximize body heat. The outfit was a fraternity boy's worst nightmare, but on Hanson it looked great; not just because he had a perfect physique, but because he was completely comfortable and at ease with himself. He didn't care what other people thought about him. He spoke only when he had something interesting to say. Otherwise he was quiet and was content to be quiet.

Hanson was everything Richard wanted to be: the strong, silent type. Richard was relatively secure with his appearance and with whom he was as a person. But for the most part he was still too immature and at war with himself to compete with Hanson in any category.

Richard's gaze swung to a dark small figure leaning against the stairwell that led to the upstairs of the next townhouse. The figure was wearing a hat pulled down over his face, but he was still familiar. Curious, Richard approached and soon recognized the face of Joe Sebastian.

Joe saw that Richard was staring at him and the two froze five yards from each other, not sure what move to make. Richard made the decision and spoke.

"Hey Joe," he said quietly. "You want a beer?"

"No thanks," Joe said in a low, defeated voice.

Richard knew Joe had been to hell and back since August. The police had drained the lake, ransacked Joe's apartment, held him in custody on a trumped-up charge that was now dismissed, and used his name freely and liberally as their sacrificial lamb to the national media by calling him their "main suspect." In the end they found no concrete evidence that he had anything to do with the five students who were murdered. The police were now claiming that it was all "just a hunch that was blown out of proportion by the media."

Joe was a free man with no criminal record, but he might as well have been dead because the name "Joe Sebastian" was synonymous with "serial killer" around Arboretum—at least until the real McCoy was found. Richard felt sorry for Joe, and thought he got a raw deal.

"How are you holding up?" Richard asked.

"I'm doing all right."

"Look. I want you to know that we stood up for you as much as we could. I don't know if it did any good, though," Richard said, sounding apologetic.

"You guys were fine," he said. "I'm just exhausted now."

"What are you gonna do now?" Richard asked.

"I gotta get out of here. I'm leaving very soon for Kentucky."

"What's up there?"

"My uncle raises horses outside Louisville," he said. Richard winced when he mentioned the town. It was the night's first reminder that his girlfriend—a native of Louisville—was at some other party.

Joe continued, "He said he'd put me to work up there on his farm until things died down. Hopefully, they'll catch this guy and my life can get back to normal. I'd like to go back to school some day."

"Here?" Richard asked. He realized it was a dumb question as soon as it came out of his mouth.

"No," he said calmly. Richard was relieved that he wasn't annoyed with the question. "I'll probably save some money from the farm work and transfer to Kentucky or Louisville. I should be able to save something, seein' as how I'll have no social life and I'll be getting 10 bucks an hour on the farm."

"Not bad; sounds like you got your shit together."

"Hey do me a favor," Joe said. "If anyone asks, even the other guys, don't tell them where I'm going. I really need some peace and quiet."

"Sure, Joe. I understand."

The journalist in Richard wanted to know if he *had* asked out all those girls, like the police were saying. But he bit his tongue and didn't let it out. There was an awkward moment of silence that signaled the end of the conversation. Joe initiated the termination.

"Well, I better finish packing and take off," he said. "Right...Hey Joe," Richard called as Joe was turning away. "I know you're a little apprehensive about coming out into the light right now. But if you want, I'll bring you a beer if you're thirsty."

"No thanks," answered Joe, who was now just a shadow in the darkness of the backyard staircase that led to the top floor of his former townhouse. "With my luck, I'll drink that beer and get charged with drunk driving tonight. I've spent enough senseless nights in jail. I don't need another."

"Right. . . Hey Joe," he called as the shadow turned back again. "Do you think you'll ever come back to Arboretum?" Richard's curiosity got the better of him again.

There was a pause and then the answer from the shadow came. "Never."

"I'm sorry," Richard said to the ground he was staring at.

"Don't be. You're a good person, Dick. Allow yourself to have a good life. You deserve it."

"You too, Joe." Richard said at the ground. He looked up and the shadow was gone.

Richard went under the staircase, where Joe had been standing to avoid the light. From his viewpoint he surveyed the area and saw that the party had grown in size since he last made an effort to notice. Richard gathered himself and moved towards Johnny and Hargrove, who were by the fire.

As he got closer he saw an attractive, statuesque woman talking to them. She was tan, about six feet tall, with long, strawberry blonde hair. Richard paused in amazement. It was Gina Moss. Richard hadn't seen her since his sophomore year. She had shorter hair then, which is what threw Richard off when he saw her by the fire. He decided she looked a lot better with her new hairdo.

Gina came to FIT the same year that Richard showed up in Arboretum. Gina came with greater credentials, though. In high school, she had recorded the fourth fastest mile in U.S. high school history: 4:38. But Gina never fit in at FIT. She was an incredible physical specimen (long legs, surprisingly well endowed for a distance runner, and naturally pretty and tanned), and was a woman who didn't need much makeup or maintenance to look beautiful. But the girl never took care of herself. She didn't shave her legs or armpits and rarely showered. She would usually unknowingly announce her presence in public with her scent, which Richard used to describe as "nature gone bad."

She had earned the nickname Crazy Gin (pronounced like the alcoholic beverage) for two reasons. First, she was legitimately insane. Gin was famous for walking around campus in track spikes and then racing in heavy-duty training shoes. That was only the tip of the iceberg. There were many other episodes that confirmed her madness.

The other half of her nickname was earned because she drank quite a bit during her two-year tenure at FIT. To boot, she slept with many athletes on the track team, including the two men she was talking to by the fire—Johnny and Hargrove. In fact, Johnny and Hargrove had sex with her at the same time. Johnny called it the "Gin sandwich."

After two years she'd had enough. She had a falling out with the women's head coach, quit the team and left Arboretum. Richard hadn't seen, heard, or thought of her since. But there she was right before his eyes—in the flesh, draining a beer. Richard approached the group at the fire.

"Gina Moss, as I live and breathe."

"Dick!" she said excitedly. She threw her arms around him and gave him a heavy whiff of her strong scent. "How are you doing?"

"I'm hanging in there."

"You still running for the Devil?"

"Yep. I'm in the fifth year of my sentence. I get paroled in May."

"Quality!" she said excitedly.

"So, what have you been doing over the past two years?" he asked.

"I've been up in D.C. I went to massage school and got into the business of massaging foreign diplomats."

"Wow! That sounds like a high paying profession," Richard said. But to him it sounded more like "the oldest profession." He imagined Gina's long legs wrapped around the head of some 60-year-old Arab sheik. Richard had a wide smile on his face from the raunchy images he was conjuring up in his head. Gina noticed the smile.

"What's so amusing?" she asked.

"Oh, nothing. What were you saying?"

"I made a lot of money from the job, but I'm sick of D.C. I needed to come back home to The Jungle."

The Jungle was the town's nickname among the students at FIT. It got the name when the school first moved from Lake City (now just another exit off I-75, about 50 miles northwest of Arboretum) because of the incredible abundance of trees. Much of the Jungle had since been cut away to make room for housing developments and the Oaks Mall, which Susan rightfully called the "Oakless."

Now The Jungle was a huge cement parking lot in front of the Wal-Mart Superstore. What a shame, Richard thought. Arboretum was a beautiful town before the land developers discovered it. He often wished he'd gone to FIT 30 years earlier. What great 20-mile runs he could have had then.

Richard was drifting in and out of his conversation with Gina. He heard her say she was going to take a look around, but he was deep in thought. Gina and Joe had given him a lot to contemplate. He only noticed she was not next to him when he took his eyes off the fire. It was 2 a.m. and most of the effects of his earlier drinking had worn off. He was immersed in so many conversations over the past few hours that he'd forgotten to drink.

That's a good thing to forget, he thought. Richard was proud to be sober so late in the evening. He looked forward to waking up without a hangover—a thought implanted in his head by his alcohol counselor after his troubled junior year. Since his counseling over a year ago, Richard looked at every party he attended as a challenge rather than a celebration. The few times in the past 15 months that he did "celebrate," he woke up the next morning regretting it. He had to hand it to himself, though, he'd only celebrated three or four times since he finished his counseling program. The other 50-something parties he'd attended, he came out victorious. Tonight, it looked like he would be declared the winner again. Richard: 50-something plus one. Beer: 3 or 4. Not a bad score. And it seemed to get easier to cut back every time.

He felt in control that night. He just wished he could control other things in his life as well as he could his alcohol intake.

Obviously one area in which he longed for more control was his relationship with Susan. Like the iceberg that awaited the arrival of the Titanic, he could see that something disastrous was going to occur. He desperately wanted to believe otherwise. But staring at the flames shooting out of the garbage can, he admitted to himself for the first time that she would never wear his ring. He could not be his true self if they were to stay together. He would end up holding in so much anger that he would surely give himself an ulcer by age 30. She was too stubborn to loosen her grip on the relationship and he was too stubborn to allow her to rule dictatorially—no matter how benevolent she tried to be. He was ruefully anticipating the day when their ship would sink. The only thing he questioned was whether or not he'd go down with the ship.

He wanted more than anything for her to be there at the party. He wanted to hold hands and stare into her eyes by the light of the fire. There was still that chance. Although she said she had other plans, Susan loved to throw an occasional change-up. She wanted to be thought of as unpredictable and mysterious. After two months though, Richard saw right through her. To him, Susan had become predictable in her unpredictability. Now her attempts to remain mysterious were just a huge annoyance to him. Although he wouldn't put money on it, he was relatively sure she wouldn't show up to Dick Stomp. He hoped he was wrong.

"Hey Dick," Gopher said, bringing Richard out of his daze. "Mad Dog's gonna read the poem. Come on in."

Mad Dog's poems were always the highlight of a party. Usually at about 2 a.m. Mad Dog would get naked and start howling. Like a mating call, this was the sign that the poem was soon to be read. His poems were read in grandiose fashion as if they were about the adventures of medieval knights. But the words were always linked to the things that dominated Mad Dog's life: drunkenness, nudity, and the everyday pain a distance runner must endure to be successful.

His poems were always written in basic four-line AABB style. Mad Dog would read the first two lines of a stanza, pause to let it sink in (and let the laughter die down), and then roll out the next two lines, to which the crowd would generally explode in laughter. The words he wrote were clever enough, but it was the delivery that made Mad Dog's poems so well received.

The apartment was quite crowded in back. Richard worked his way up to the front and saw Mad Dog howling naked on the puke couch. He saw the hard-core guys—Phil, Atlas, Jeff, Hargrove, Johnny and Gopher—begin to strip. Not wanting to be left out, Richard took his clothes off and flung them into the corner between the puke couch and the wall. The nudists cleared a space for themselves by pushing some of the clothed on-lookers back a few steps. Most of the party-goers didn't want to be too close to these crazy naked men and were more than willing to take two steps back. Once given room to operate, the seven nudists got down on their knees below Mad Dog and awaited the poem. The crowd hushed and Mad Dog began:

"We are the clickers, the rollers, the midnight controllers,
The ones with the strength, the exhaustion bestowers.
Taking on the night with no regret,
Sleeping all day after a high dice bet
We take on the world, beer after beer,
Staring death in the eyes without true fear.
Playing a hand of cards dealt in life,
We accept the madness without strife.
With high quality gas, we ride the road,
Invisible to sight and in stealth mode.
We are the few, the rare, the handpicked ones,

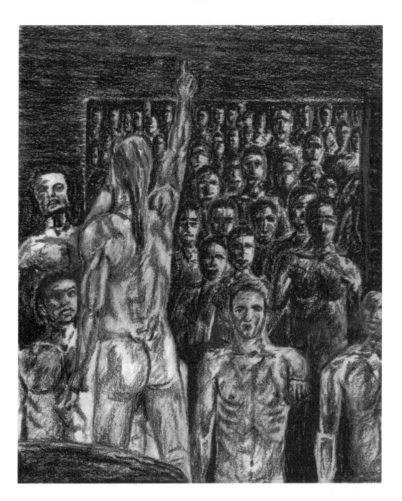

Rolling through life with double shotguns.
So beware the weak, you know your own name,
Cause we're playing the night, down the high road to fame."

The crowd responded to the poem like a good race. They cheered at every turn. They got louder on each lap. And they went into a fury as the poem and the reader rounded the corner into the homestretch and crossed the finish line. The response at the end was especially intense in the crowded living room. It reminded Richard of the response the crew of the Pequod gave Captain Ahab after his motivating speech about hunting down Moby Dick. After the poem, Richard half-expected the crowd to shout in unison a Melvillian "Huzza! Huzza!"

After a few naked kegstands, Richard put his clothes back on and went out to stare at the fire, which was now being fueled by a wooden desk that one of the neighbors had left on his porch.

At 4 a.m. a police officer came by. The party was still going strong with about 20 people still drinking and raising hell. The officer walked up to Richard, by the fire. It was their third visit of the evening.

"Excuse me. Do you live here?"

"Yes I do, officer."

"It's 4 a.m. It's time to end the party."

Richard sent the officer on his way, assuring him that the party was about over. He went inside, shut the sliding glass door and turned down the music a few notches. He looked to his right and saw Mad Dog and Gin wrestling on the puke couch, completely naked. He shook his head and smiled.

"I should have known," he whispered to himself. "The two craziest people I know. They were meant for each other."

The Morning After

At 9 a.m. Richard was awakened by the ring of the phone. "Hello."

"Hi," Susan said. "Did I wake you?"

"What do you think?" he said in a sarcastic tone. She laughed.

"I have a hangover," she said in a pouting voice. "Why don't you come over here and take care of me."

"I'd love to," he said, "but that would mean I'd actually have to get up. I'm too lazy to get up to take a piss. I'm contemplating just urinating in my bed. It wouldn't be so bad. It would feel warm for a while and I have to wash the sheets anyway." She laughed hard.

"Quit making me laugh. It hurts," she whined. "Why don't you come over here and crawl in bed and tell me all about the party. I wanna know everything," she said.

"All right," he surrendered.

"And on your way over can you pick up some orange juice?

I need juice to recover from my hangover."

"I knew there was a catch," he said.

She pleaded with him and he eventually agreed. He loved to hear her beg. And the thought of hopping in bed with her had brought all of his body parts to a rise. He was knocking on her back door 20 minutes after they hung up the phone.

"Who is it?" came the teasing voice.

In his best Brooklyn accent he said, "Yo, I got a special delivery for a Mister S. Connor."

"What is it?" she asked, curious to hear what would come out of his mouth. The New York accent turned her on.

"Yo lady, I don't know. I don't look inside da packages I deliva. I got a wife and five kids. I need dis job. But if I had to guess, I'd say it was a box a rubbas."

He heard her laughing loudly as she unlocked the door. She greeted him, clothed in a smile and nothing else. He greeted her with the orange juice.

Richard poured two glasses of O.J. and put them next to the bed. He stripped and hopped in next to her. Susan picked up her glass, took some aspirin, and laid back down. She turned toward Richard and said in that sultry voice, "Now, tell me everything."

Richard told her most of what he'd experienced the night before. He left out the morose thoughts by the fire.

6

Motivation

It was 3 a.m. on the morning of November 3rd—a Monday. Richard had just watched the replay of Penn State's upset win over Notre Dame in his living room. In eight hours he would hear the gun sound to start the SEC Cross Country Championships.

There was something about the conference meet that boiled Richard's blood more than anything. He'd run in larger meets. He'd been to five NCAA championship meets. But none of those meets could hold a candle to the intensity of the SEC meet, whether it be cross country, indoor or outdoor track.

When Richard came to school he was told that the top priority at FIT was to win the conference. A national championship would be nice, but a conference championship was a must. To some, the priority of a smaller championship over a larger one didn't make sense. But to Richard it was crystal clear. He saw it as the difference between a fist fight in a bar with a stranger, and a fist fight with your own brother. A fight with the stranger is forgotten a few days later. A serious brawl with a sibling is a lot more deep-seated and is often never forgotten.

Richard didn't know about other conferences, but in the SEC, the conference championships were an all-out family feud. This added intensity helped keep Richard awake throughout the night. He looked at his watch and felt his pulse—97 beats per minute.

"If you don't get some sleep, Richard, you'll run like shit for sure," he told himself.

But giving himself sleep ultimatums never worked. So he took a deep breath and resigned himself to the fact that he would get only a couple of hours sleep, if he was lucky. It was at times like this that he asked himself the question every athlete has to ask, "Why do I put myself through this hell?"

Richard, like every other athlete, competed for a reason. When things get tough, it is that reason an athlete looks to for the motivation needed to succeed. For some, the reason is money. Others are addicted to winning. Some live for the thrill of toeing the line and competing against great athletes, even if they're not at that level. And still others do it to please someone else—usually a parent.

When athletes experience "burnout," the driving reason that made them go out and work every day is gone. The reason is no longer sufficient to get them to work as hard as they did before. They either have to find a new reason to compete or they quit, or—even worse—they continue to compete, but at a level that is embarrassing to themselves and to those who know what they are capable of. This happened to some of Richard's high school competitors—guys who he'd have to outkick to beat, he was now lapping.

Some people talk about the diminishing physical skills of older athletes as a reason why they retire. The loss of motivation, Richard thought, is the biggest reason athletes at all levels call it quits. It would eventually be his reason for quitting.

There's only one way to explain why Jim Brown and John McEnroe quit their respective sports in their late 20's while Gordie Howe played hockey into his 50's. For Brown and McEnroe, domination in their sports extinguished their fires in the prime of their career. There were no more worlds to conquer, and the motivation was lost for them.

Both attempted comebacks. Brown's occurred over 15 years after his initial retirement and ended in the L.A. Raiders' training camp. Neither were able to reach the level they were at when they first retired. On the other hand, Gordie Howe never lost the fire to play hockey even though he was 20 years past his physical prime when he finally retired.

Richard admired Howe and Jimmy Connors, who played tennis past the age of 40, because their motivation came not from reaching the top, but from the joy of competing in the games they loved. It was this pure love of sport, this positive energy, that enabled them to keep their motivation.

Richard knew it was only athletes with this positive energy who endured. His own energy was completely negative. He knew he was motivated not by the love of his sport, but rather an inner rage that burned hotter than coal in a locomotive engine.

And part of this rage, he knew, harkened back to experiences in his own life, experiences which exposed him to the cruelty which people are capable of inflicting. Whenever he questioned his own motivation, he often flashed back to one particular relationship in his young life—the Brendles.

When he was five his family moved from their Brooklyn apartment to a new detached house in Long Island. While it was only a 30-mile move, it was a universe apart for Richard. He did take to the physical surroundings quickly—the house had a nice lawn in the front and back yard, a street he could play in, and a bedroom three times the size of his old room.

But Long Island also had Kevin and Kenny Brendle. The Brendle brothers were Richard's first friends in the new neighborhood. Kevin was a year older and Kenny two years younger, and for a few years, the three got along fine. Even the parents became friends—for a while. But without explaining why, Richard's parents stopped socializing with the Brendles after a couple of years. They never told Richard he couldn't play with the boys, and he never asked what brought about the change. But he remembered noticing.

Richard and Kevin became best friends. Kenny tailed along often, but, as the youngster, he was more tolerated than accepted. Kenny was the baggage that came with Kevin. Time to themselves, without Kenny, was rare, because Kenny would usually annoy his mother until she commanded, "Kevin, take Kenny with you," or "Kevin, let Kenny play with you." During the summer, their main refuge from Kenny was the local summer band program at the elementary school, where they both played the trumpet.

The Kevin-Richard relationship all changed when Kevin started junior high school at Fresh Meadows Junior/Senior High. Richard detected changes the summer before. Kevin started picking on Kenny with greater frequency and venom than he had previously. And he began to distance himself from Richard.

A few weeks before school started, Richard came calling for Kevin. Mrs. Brendle—who Richard feared more than anyone on earth—came to the door and shouted in her cigarette-scratchy voice, "Kevin, it's Richard." "Tell him to go away," came back a voice from the dark. It was Kevin's voice, which was changing as fast as his attitude.

Richard stared, dumbfounded and humiliated, at Mrs. Brendle, who regarded him with a smirk on her face. "You heard

him, Richard," she said. "He doesn't want to play with you today." She closed the door with the 11-year-old standing there
in shock.

Richard ran home in tears. Kevin was his first friend, his
best friend, and his only friend within walking distance of his
house—a crucial matter to a grade schooler. Now that friendship was suddenly no more.

Richard didn't have a lot of friends. Furthermore, many of
the kids he knew from school and his soccer team picked on
him because he was small, gullible, sensitive, Jewish, and he
didn't defend himself well, either physically or verbally. He was
pretty much an outsider during those formative years, which
was one reason why Kevin's friendship had been so important
to him.

All this caused profound changes in Richard. He became
reluctant to trust anyone. He also learned to keep his sensitivi-
ties inside and to develop a sharp tongue, ready to strike out at
anyone who tried to get at him. He figured if he could deliver a
comeback that was cleverer and harsher than the original insult, he wouldn't look like such an easy target and he wouldn't
be messed with so often.

It was bad enough that Kevin Brendle had cast him off as a
friend, but that was far from the end of their relationship. As a
junior high student who couldn't be seen dead with an elementary school kid, Kevin now felt it was his duty to pick on Richard.

Richard didn't stand much of a chance. Kevin was signifi-
cantly bigger and stronger. Richard had always been faster and
quicker, but now that Kevin was reaching puberty, little Richard Dubin couldn't outrun him as easily.

When they were at different schools, the abuse was limited. Kevin was on the junior high soccer team and didn't get
home till near dark. He didn't have much time to pick on Richard except for the weekends.

But when Richard entered junior high, the abuse escalated.
In the halls, at band practice, on the playing fields—no arena
was safe from Kevin. And teachers and coaches were conveniently oblivious.

Kevin's standard threat was: "I'm going to kick your fuckin'
ass." "You'd better be careful walking home today," he'd shout.
"I'm looking for you, Dubin."

Kevin wasn't just talking for the sake of hearing his own

voice. Most bullies want an audience of peers when they issue their threats.

Walking home from school was always an ordeal for Richard. Kevin never waited for him, but their paths were the same. If they happened to spot each other, it was usually a contest to see if Richard could make it to his front door before being pummeled. Fortunately, he usually made it.

So, Richard's running ability developed out of a necessity to stay alive. When the soccer team had to run a mile around the school track in under eight minutes—or be forced to do it again the following week—Richard "jogged" in in under six minutes, finishing 30 seconds ahead of the second-place runner. When Brendle struggled in in 8:10, he gasped and said, "Hey, Dubin, let me borrow your lungs next week."

They were the first civil words Kevin had spoken to Richard since that day at the Brendle front door. They were the only civil words he would ever say to him again.

Still, Richard's running prowess must have impressed Kevin somewhat, because although the harassment and bullying never stopped, there were very few beatings after that.

When Kenny came to junior high school, he tried to adopt the bullying act as well, but was not as successful. With Kevin in tenth grade and on the junior varsity soccer team and the high school band, Richard didn't have to focus on avoiding him as much. He decided he'd taken it from the older brother long enough, and wasn't about to take it from a seventh grader.

So, before Kenny got the first bile completely out of his mouth in the locker room, Richard put a finger in his face (in front of the whole soccer team) and said, "You'd better keep your trap shut, Kenny, before I send you home bawling to Mama, like we used to. And don't think your big brother's gonna come and save you either, because he hates you worse than I do."

That preemptive strike pretty much defused Kenny. Though they still fought occasionally that year, Richard had the upper hand every time. Though Kenny outweighed Richard, he didn't know how to throw it around like his brother. And he wasn't as mean or smart as Kevin.

Showing the Brendles that he was not an insignificant wimp was an important motivating factor when Richard went out for the track team later on, and he had to thank them for unwittingly pushing him toward the success he did achieve as a distance runner.

Being bullied and left out as a child was not the only flame that burned in Richard's stomach. Disbelievers fueled his anger as much as the bullies.

Richard remembered very little of his years on the junior high track team. But two quotes stuck in his mind from eighth grade that he'd never forget as long as he lived. One came from Jason Mandel, a sprinter on the team, at Mandel's July 4th barbecue.

"Face it Richard," he said. "I'm a great sprinter. You're just an average distance runner."

The other came from the junior high coach after Richard lost to a more physically mature teammate named Jimmy Ingenito.

"Richard, you're never going to beat Jimmy," the coach said.

Ingenito made all-conference in the two-mile his senior year. Mandel made all-conference in the 200. Richard finished high school as the 10th fastest two-miler in U.S. prep history.

Richard didn't hold any bitterness toward the people who'd made those statements, he just remembered them. He remained friends with Ingenito. And he was so close with Mandel, in fact, that Richard served as his best man at his wedding. Richard never spoke a kind word to the junior high coach again, though. But that was not because of his statement; he just didn't like the man.

There were other things said about Richard in high school, but none were remembered as vividly as those gibes. They became his inner battle cry during his high school career.

His high school coach would always make sure that negative comments found their way back to Richard's ear, even if he had to embellish them a bit. He knew what motivated Richard to excel.

"Tell him what he can't do and he'll work twice as hard to prove you wrong," he once privately told Richard's father.

Richard was thinking about going away to college at the start of his senior year, but only within a few hours driving distance of home. Penn State, Boston University, and Syracuse appealed to him early on. When he found out about a coach's comment through Devlin, who was recruiting him at the time, he decided he needed to go much farther away.

Walt O'Leary, the St. John's track coach, had wanted Richard in a big way. But when he found out that Richard was looking to leave Long Island, he instituted a smear campaign against him. O'Leary would denigrate Richard to any college coach who mentioned his name. He would tell potential recruiters how Richard was impossible to coach and how he liked to smoke marijuana.

None of these statements were completely false. Richard would often question his coach's workouts, although he respected his coach and always did the workouts to the best of his ability. Richard had also smoked pot back in the ninth and tenth grades. But he quit when he started taking his running somewhat seriously.

His quitting marijuana also coincided with a bad experience in which he unknowingly smoked a joint laced with LSD. Richard hallucinated that he was looking at himself being buried. The experience scared him so badly that he didn't take a puff of anything until his sophomore year in college.

A lot of recruiters were scared off by what O'Leary had said. Devlin was not. He called Richard to hear his side of the story. He told Devlin how O'Leary started spreading rumors after Richard turned him down. Devlin seemed impressed by Richard's honesty. Richard respected Devlin for not rejecting him out of hand. He was apprehensive about going to school 1,100 miles from home. But Long Island seemed to have as much animosity toward Richard as he had toward it. He decided to go to FIT in January—three months before the earliest signing day.

When the bullies' effects wore off in high school, it was the naysayers and the underestimators who kept Richard motivated to run fast. And to Richard, those skeptics seemed to be everywhere—in New York, in Arboretum, in the stands at every track meet he ran. He *had* to show them all. And when he ran poorly, he would tear himself apart inside because he had temporarily proved the naysayers right.

It was midway through his senior year in high school that Richard heard on the radio about a car crashing into a telephone poll. There were no passengers and the driver was killed instantly. Drunk driving was suspected to be the cause of the incident. The driver's name was Kevin Brendle of Fresh Meadows, N.Y. Many friends and well-wishers attended the funeral.

Richard was not one of them. He wondered how many people at the funeral really liked Kevin while he was alive, how many there were really sad that he was gone. "Kevin got his," Richard would say to himself. But deep down, he really wished he'd had the guts to take a full back swing with his trumpet and plant it in Kevin's face while he was alive.

Morning Conversation

At 6:15 in the morning, Richard did what he had done before so many important meets—he called home. In crisis situations like this, his father could always calm him down. He figured he'd better call now before his father left for work.

Richard didn't understand how a few moments of conversation with his father could restore his serenity. Maybe it was his deep voice. Maybe it was the fact that he never knew what race his son was running, and therefore, it must not be the life-and-death situation Richard made it out to be. At times like these, though, Richard didn't care about understanding, he just wanted the cure.

"Hello, Dad?"

"Hey," he said in his I-just-woke-up voice. "I guess you're nervous about some race."

"Yeah. We got the conference meet today at eleven."

"Oh. That's nice. Are you ready to run?"

"I think so. I mean, yeah."

"OK, then. So what are you nervous about?"

"I don't really know. I guess I get so worked up about kicking ass that I can't settle down. I want to win as an individual. But more importantly I want to run well and help the team. I want to run well so badly that the thought of running slow keeps me up.

"I'm not sure," Richard continued. "All I know right now is that I'm in a living hell. I couldn't sleep at all last night."

"Listen, Richard," his father said softly and slowly like a good hypnotist. "Nothing is worth what you're putting yourself through. Nothing. You're still going to have people that love you no matter what place you finish. As for the team, you can only control what you do. I know you'd like to control what the other guys do, but you can't. Nothing you do will make your teammates run faster or your competitors run slower. The only thing you can do is your best, which you and everyone else knows you'll give.

"Look," he continued. "You still have time to get some rest. If you don't feel tired, go out and run a couple of miles, take a shower, and take a nap."

"Running?" Richard asked. "You think I should go running now?"

"Sure. You run how many miles a week?"

"Eighty."

"Two miles shouldn't hurt you, Richard."

"All right, I'll try it," Richard said. But suddenly he wanted to do nothing but sleep.

"Listen, I have to get to work. So take care. Good luck. And hey, take it easy on yourself."

"OK, Pop."

"And give us a call tonight to let us know how you made out, OK?"

"All right. I'll talk to you later. Bye."

He hung up the phone and passed out on the puke couch.

Warm-up

Richard was awakened at 8:30 by Jeff, Gopher and Mad Dog, who were stirring around in the kitchen, preparing for the race they each had to run.

"Good morning," Jeff said when he saw Richard begin to wake. "You sleep well last night, Champ?"

"What do you think?" he responded rhetorically.

"How many hours?" Gopher asked. Richard would be asked that same question at least 10 times throughout the day.

"About two," he responded.

"Damn," Gopher said. "I don't understand how you can run on that kind of sleep."

"Adrenaline and talent," Richard said. "That's all you need."

Richard felt pretty relaxed and refreshed from his nap. People used to laugh when they saw the puke couch. But anyone who dared to lay down on it felt drowsy upon contact. The puke couch was ugly, but it was undeniably comfortable and great for napping.

He went into the kitchen and fixed himself two cinnamon raisin bagels with margarine. Most mornings he put cream cheese on his bagels, but margarine was a safer, more easily digestible alternative before a race. He wolfed them both down.

At 9:30 he was all fueled up. He went to his room and began assembling the racing items he'd bring to the course—singlet and spikes were already in the spikebag. He put on his warm-up shirt, racing shorts, racing socks and training shoes.

Even with two pit stops at home since 9:30, he was sure he'd have to go again after his two-mile warm-up. He loathed the thought of going in a stinky, slimy, hot Port-a-John at the course when he lived less than a half-mile away. But sometimes one has to accept a little less quality in exchange for greater convenience.

He got his things together and walked over to the golf course with his roommates. Nothing was said on the walk over; if there were words spoken, Richard didn't hear them. Those who ran with him knew the futility of attempting conversation before a race.

The crew got to the meeting area at 10:10—an hour and five minutes before race time. Richard felt relaxed, he even had a little smile on his face. He was in the best shape of his life. He was ready to go. He was confident. And when Richard was relaxed and confident, he usually did great things.

An anxious Devlin walked up to Richard and asked, "You ready to go, Stud?"

After the first few words came out of his mouth, Richard could tell that Devlin had foregone the tobacco he chewed on a daily basis for a roll of chewable antacid tablets. Such was the grip any SEC meet had on Devlin.

"Ready to complete the mission, Boss."

"Glad to hear it," Devlin said. "You get any sleep last night?"

"I could ask you the same question," said Richard, who was beginning to grow tired of the same pre-race question.

"Yeah, well, it don't matter how tired I am. I ain't gotta run five miles."

"Praise the Lord," Richard smart-assed. He could get away with this kind of talk before a big meet, but only if he ran well. If he didn't, Devlin would be sure to remind him of that comment as soon as he crossed the finish line.

By 10:20 the entire cast was present: the four Clubhouse residents, Anthony, Dante, and James Bache, a freshman who was beginning to show promise.

Bache was an underdeveloped 5-8, 120-pounder with brown hair that was usually uncombed in a mop top. He was a quiet, nondescript 4:30 miler from a tiny high school in the Florida Panhandle. He walked on to the team and struggled in the back of the pack—along with Richard—in the early season work-outs.

Bache, however, was a prizefighter's worst nightmare; he was one of those guys who would get knocked down but could be counted on to never get counted out. Eventually he'd wear you down. Bache got hammered in almost every workout, but he kept on showing up. And, as the season progressed, he began to find ways to beat some of the guys who he couldn't hang with earlier in the year.

Little by little, with much encouragement from Richard and a couple of others, he worked his way up to the seventh position at the FIT Invitational—the last race before the SEC meet—and earned a permanent spot on the team.

Richard loved Bache because he was Richard's embodiment of what athletics are all about: shut up, work hard, don't give up, and eventually (hopefully) you will be rewarded for your efforts.

"You can have your spoiled-rotten talented athletes," Richard told Devlin one day after practice. "You give me seven James Baches, I'll take on the world."

Devlin had no respect for walk-ons. He had even cut Bache earlier in the season, but the kid showed up to practice the next day as if nothing had changed. Devlin wasn't even sure he liked the idea that the kid openly defied him by showing up to practice after being cut, not to mention having the audacity to beat some of his scholarship athletes. Devlin laughed at Richard's enthusiasm toward Bache and the other walk-ons—which probably explained why there were so many talented underachievers in the FIT program.

As the group of seven went out for their two-mile warm-up, Richard looked around at some of the other teams jogging. Viewing the grounds, he couldn't spot Tennessee or Kentucky—the favorites. The hope began to rise in his heart that maybe they just forgot to show up. But he quickly squelched that ridiculous thought. He knew his main competitors were not only present, but were going to run fast. Therefore, he would too.

This fiery thought settled his queasy stomach. The idea of a battle to the ultimate end, as in medieval times, helped Richard lock into the tenacious attitude he needed to run well. The thought of running till he dropped from exhaustion was somehow comforting. He may lose the big race, but no one would ever doubt his fighting spirit.

No one really ever had doubts about that part of Richard. Even so, this very doubt kept him awake many a night, questioning himself. All his teammates understood that in the end Richard would give his all—which is all you can ask of any athlete. Everyone was positive of this, except Richard. But as the warm-up progressed, Richard became more secure in the fact that he would run well and, more importantly, that he would give every ounce of energy to the cause.

The warm-up ended as the team sat down to stretch at the start of the horse shoe loop—about a quarter-mile from the race starting line. As Richard was stretching he saw Tennessee, the team favorite, jog by. Tennessee's Terry Johnson, the individual favorite, looked confident to the point of cockiness. Richard wondered if that look was hiding a nervousness below, like the one he currently felt, or if he were truly overconfident. Richard hoped it was the latter. It would be much easier to sneak up and surprise Johnson and his team, than to face a mentally prepared Tennessee squad.

They'd won the title three years in a row. Johnson was the only team member left who'd been through their last loss, which was due mostly to overconfidence as well. No other current Tennessee team member had yet to experience losing the SEC Cross Country Championship.

Teams have a way of taking things for granted when they haven't lost in a while. A winning team may start thinking they can't lose, and whether they realize it or not, they stop giving that small amount of extra effort in practice, which is what took them to the top.

While Richard felt Johnson's teammates were possible candidates for the overconfidence syndrome, he knew that Johnson was not. One of the reasons Johnson won practically every race he ran was because he never took anyone or any race for granted.

In conversations with Johnson, Richard realized the profound impact that SEC loss four years ago had on him. Johnson finished second in that race behind only Hargrove and did all he could to help his team win. But Johnson could see the pre-race cockiness then in his teammates—who'd won the previous eight SEC titles. After the loss, Johnson vowed to himself to never let the overconfidence bug affect him.

Johnson had a certain ethereal knowledge that only the great ones have. It was a feeling that was developed over years of successful racing. This attitude said simply, "It's time to run fast. Therefore I *will* run fast." Johnson didn't stay up nights worrying about whether or not he would run well. That fact was as inevitable as the rotating earth. And if he lost, which was rare, it wasn't because he had a bad day; it was because another great runner with that same confidence had an even better day.

That confidence is a tremendous advantage, and something that every runner striving for greatness yearns to have. Some even take performance-enhancing and life-threatening drugs to achieve that peace of mind. Richard would gladly have given up a limb to have it.

Johnson would run well, no doubt. But five score in a cross country meet, and the candidates for the other four positions on the Tennessee squad were questionable. Richard took some comfort in that.

Tennessee and Kentucky weren't the only powerful squads in the field. Defending national champions Arkansas would also be running.

Looking down the the roster for Arkansas could be an intimidating experience—Olympic and World Championship finalists from Canada, Ireland and Great Britain, as well as some fine American talent. Unfortunately for Arkansas, three of their top four runners were coming off injuries that had kept them from competing all season. Word had it that they were starting to get fit and would compete at the NCAA Championships. But their coach decided to hold them out of the SEC race as a precaution. Only the Brit, David Allen, would compete this week.

With all their guys healthy, they would be a strong favorite to take the conference and national titles. Without them, Arkansas was merely a better-than-average squad.

Richard figured the Arkansas coach didn't want his world-class studs to experience the rigors of the FIT home course in their first competition of the season.

"Smart move," thought Richard.

When Richard and his teammates finished stretching, they laced up their spikes, and walked over to the starting line to do some pre-race 100-meter strides to loosen the legs. He ran his strides at about race pace, much slower than the all-out sprints his teammates were doing. That was partly out of pre-race nerves and partly because Richard started all cross country races in the middle to the back of the pack.

His starts always worried Devlin because he was typically far behind the leaders—and many of the joggers—at the half-mile mark. But he felt better than just about everyone ahead of him, and would pass most of the quick starters within the next mile or two, leaving still more than half the race to go.

Richard had just finished a stride and was walking back to the starting line when Devlin called the team over for his final words. As he walked back, he caught someone's eye. It was his longtime friend Jim Bird, whom he jokingly called "The Shadow." Bird got the nickname because, while Richard was a more talented athlete on the track, he couldn't shake Bird—or beat him—in cross country. Their rivalry was a friendly one, though. And if Richard's Aggies were to lose on that day, he would rather have it be at the hands of Bird and Kentucky, than to Johnson and Tennessee. Richard was sure that Bird felt the same way.

The Aggies gathered in a tight circle behind the starting line. Each member put his hand in the center. Richard hated these tense moments, being next to these six other sweaty, smelly, nervous runners, and a coach who was as nervous as all of them put together. Why couldn't they just leave him alone and let him do his thing?

He longed for the day when it would just be him running for himself, without the expectations of coaches and teammates. Without the worries of scoring points at a conference or national meet. Just running for himself. "Team Richard," he would call it. When he could have that freedom, that's when he figured running would feel more like a passion, instead of what it currently felt like standing in that huddle—a job that was putting him through college.

"All right, boys," Devlin said in the tight huddle. "This is it. Fight for every position out there. Someone's gonna walk away with that trophy up at the golfhouse. I'd kinda like to just walk it down the road to my office. But it ain't up to me.

You're here. You gotta run. You might as well win this sombitch and send'em home cryin'. All right, on three let's hear it. One, two, three." And the team shouted, "F-I-T! FIGHT!" in unison. Richard shouted nothing.

He tuned out the entire speech and kept repeating the same sentence in his head over and over. "Just get me to the line." The mantra referred to the starting line. He always believed that once he was at the starting line, everything else would take care of itself. After his teammates gave the shout, he got his wish.

The Aggies lined up in Box #3, their assigned position along the starting line. John Jenkins, the ancient official, appeared in the middle of the field about 30 yards in front of the starting line.

Jenkins had walked by Richard earlier. Just as he'd done before so many other races, Jenkins gave him the standard wink, which was his version of "Good Luck." Richard liked the wink because it was one little facial movement that said a lot. Besides "Good Luck," the wink said, "I have confidence that you'll come through because you're a winner."

The beauty was that there were no words spoken. Jenkins understood how Richard worked before a race and knew exactly how to get his message across where it would best be understood and appreciated. Richard and Jenkins were on the same wave length, which is one reason why they were such good friends. Over the years, Jenkins had become Richard's lone father figure in Arboretum.

"All right, gentlemen," Jenkins said into his megaphone. "I'm going to say 'Runners set,' and then I'll fire the gun. After I fire the gun I'm going to run on over here to your right. Since ya'll are running to the left you shouldn't have a problem avoiding me. But just in case I have a heart attack along the way, just hop over me." The crowd, and even most of the runners, started laughing. "On a serious note, if there's a spill within the first 100 yards, I'll fire the gun a couple of times and we'll bring it back and try again. You got about one minute till the start, so let's get ready. Good luck, gentlemen."

Richard lightly shook his legs to keep them loose and to harmlessly work off some of his nervous energy. He shook hands with Anthony.

"This is it, Dick," Anthony said. "Let's try to close our careers the same way we opened them."

Richard nodded his approval, thinking to himself, "If you can put it together for one race, Anthony, maybe we can do it." He shook hands with each member of his team except Mad Dog, who was busy doing one last stride.

"All right, gentlemen, get to your box," Jenkins said. Mad Dog ran back to the line and hopped in the box. Richard stood with Anthony on his right and Mad Dog on his left. "Runners set. . . BANG!"

The Race

Richard started the race in the middle of the pack and felt relatively comfortable as he rounded the first corner onto the horseshoe loop. By the half-mile point he'd moved up and settled into fifth place. Only Mad Dog and some unknown guys from the University of Georgia were ahead of him. The pace was slow, but he didn't mind. A slow race was to his advantage, since he had the most finishing speed among any of the legitimate contenders in the field.

The Georgia unknowns led the race through the mile in 5:05, which was about ten seconds slower than Richard thought they were running. Richard heard the time at the mile mark and looked to the right at his friend Jim "Shadow" Bird. Bird responded with a shrug and said, "Guess it's a four-mile race, now."

While Richard didn't mind a slow pace, he didn't want to jog for the first mile because the favorites might respond with alarm and take off like the start of another race. Those fears came true when Mad Dog took the lead and stepped up the pace drastically. He quickly opened a 10-meter lead on the field. Race co-favorites, Johnson and David Allen, were both jogging in back of Richard for the first mile. Together, as if they'd rehearsed it a hundred times, they surged past Richard and made up the gap. It looked so easy to Richard, who looked at Bird, and nodded. The two took off and caught up to the lead pack, though not nearly as smoothly as Johnson and Allen had done.

Richard settled into the back of that pack. The group went through two miles in 9:55—a 4:50 second mile. They stayed together for another half-mile when Johnson threw in a surge up the first huge hill. Allen, Bird and Mad Dog went with him.

Richard didn't have the strength, and watched as his hopes of an SEC individual title pulled away. By the time Richard got to the three-mile mark, the lead pack had opened up 10 seconds on him.

Richard's three-mile time was 14:45—another 4:50 - which meant that the leaders ran 4:40. His only hope was that the lead pack would die. But Richard knew that Johnson and Allen were too good to fall apart. There was no way, he thought, that anyone in the lead pack—and probably the whole field—felt as awful as he did at three miles. He was dying and there was little he could do to stop it.

But just as Richard began to feel sorry for himself, Anthony came up on him, patted him on the butt, and said, "Let's go. Stick with me."

Richard looked behind and saw a multitude of Tennessee and Kentucky runners who were closing in on him. The thought of being responsible for losing the SEC title scared Richard enough to put him back in the race. He tucked in behind Anthony and found some new life in his legs. If we have three in the top six, we've got a shot, he thought.

As they went around the horseshoe loop the second time, Richard saw that Johnson, Allen, and Bird had opened a gap on Mad Dog. Richard, with Anthony still leading the way, went through four miles in 19:50—a 5:05 mile.

As Richard ascended the hill at the end of the horseshoe loop, he saw Johnson and Allen descending the hill. Richard estimated they were about 25 seconds ahead of him. They had opened up about 8-10 seconds on Bird and 15 seconds on Mad Dog, both of whom were slowly coming back to Richard and Anthony.

Down the backside of the hill they went, Anthony smoothly extended his legs and opened up a small lead on Richard, whose arms and legs were flailing out of control. But for each downhill where Anthony excelled, there was an uphill where Richard made up the gap. And after they ran up the huge hill for the last time, Richard had taken a slight lead on Anthony.

At the top of the hill, Richard stopped for a full second, bent over, vomited the remains of his breakfast, and began his descent down the hill. About halfway down the hill, Anthony passed him. But this time Richard made a concerted effort to stay close to him. There was only one uphill and one downhill left, both about 200 meters each. If he could open up enough of a lead on the uphill, he could hold off Anthony on the last downhill.

At the bottom of the hill, they rounded a tree by the starting line. Richard, who had been feeling dizzy since he threw up, was having trouble keeping his balance and almost tripped over a tree root. "Just another quarter-mile," he told himself. "Then you can collapse."

Richard put his head down and concentrated on his running form to help him make it uphill. Without noticing, he passed Anthony and Mad Dog before he made the left turn at the start of the horseshoe and began the 200-meter downhill sprint to the finish line. On the downhill he looked up and saw Shadow Bird 50 yards ahead.

"I can catch him! I can catch him!" he told himself and began a wild, out of control kick down the hill. Richard was gaining ground on Bird with every step, but so was Anthony. In the last 30 yards, Richard's eyes were closed, his body on autopilot, knowing exactly how far it was to the finish line. Richard's body dove at the finish line, taking out Bird, Anthony, some officials, and the wood stakes that were holding up one whole side of the finish chute.

When the trainers got to him, Richard was only partially conscious and mumbling some words that no one could make out. His heart rate was well over 200 beats per minute. They dragged him to the medical area, laid him down, put a needle in his forearm, and attached an I.V. bag filled with water and electrolytes. He came around after about five minutes and sat up.

"You all right there, buddy?" asked one of the trainers.

"Yeah, I suppose," he said in a groggy voice, like he'd been asleep for eight hours.

"You had a nice little wreck there at the finish line. Does anything hurt?"

"Everything hurts, right now."

"Well, you smashed into those wood sticks at the finish line pretty good. You remember that?"

"Not at the moment."

"All right, then. You've got some good scrapes from that fall, but that's no big deal. If you have any other pains that are out of the ordinary, you be sure to come by and see us tomorrow. I don't want you runnin' around with any broken bones, OK?"

"Yep," Richard said. The trainer removed the I.V. needle from his arm, gave him two cups of water and sent him away.

He walked over to where the rest of the team was recovering. He looked around at his teammates and some of the other teams. All these runners: some sweaty and exhausted, others on the ground writhing in pain. They looked like a bunch of soldiers who'd just been through a great battle in the Civil War. In a way, they had been.

"Where's Devlin?" Richard asked.

"He's up at the golfhouse trying to figure out our score," Dante said.

"How'd you do?" he asked Dante.

"Shitty. I got a cramp at three miles. And I faded."

"Oh, no," Richard said. No matter how well Mad Dog, Anthony and Richard did, they needed strong performances from Jeff and Dante at the fourth and fifth positions. With a bad performance by Dante, it was over.

"Fortunately," Dante continued, "I wasn't fifth man."

"What? Who was, Gopher?" Richard said. Even worse, he thought. The man who can't stand pain was our fifth man. We're third place for sure.

"No," Dante said. "Bache was fifth man."

Richard's jaw dropped. The gutsy freshman who was cut midway through the season was now fifth man.

"Unbelievable," he said finally. They may have had no chance of winning with Bache, but Richard felt better about losing with him, than with Gopher as fifth man.

Richard walked up to Bache and said, "Good job."

"Thanks," he said quietly.

"What place did you get?"

"Don't know."

"Does anyone know what place they got?"

"We went four, five, and six," said Anthony.

"We did, huh. Well, who was what?" Richard asked.

"You were fourth, I was fifth, Mike was sixth," Anthony said. He always referred to Mad Dog by the name his mother gave him.

"I guess that means we didn't get Bird."

"Nope," Anthony said.

"Well, we got three down," Richard said. "Does anybody else know what place they got?"

There was a collective negative head shake from Dante, Jeff,

Bache and Gopher. Devlin came jogging back to the group with an anxious look on his face.

"All right, boys," Devlin said, out of breath after his brief run. "Let's get our stuff and head on up to the golfhouse."

"What's goin' on Devlin? How'd we do?" Richard asked. The other team members chimed in too, wanting to know the results of their efforts.

"They don't know. It's close," he said.

"Close for what? Second? Third? What?" Richard said.

"They don't know. That's why I want all you guys up there."

"Well, what's up with that shit?" Richard said, now getting irritated with Devlin's sudden evasiveness.

"What's up," Devlin snapped back, "is that your little dive into the chute screwed up the whole scoring system. You know that in an NCAA cross country race, you're supposed to go all the way through the chute, not around the side? They could have disqualified you for that."

"Fuck that," Richard responded, defensively. "They're not gonna disqualify me. Not now. Not at home."

"Well you're right about the home part," Devlin said. "Because if your old friend John Jenkins wasn't the head official, you probably would have been. About 15 minutes ago you had two coaches screamin' at him to DQ you. But he said you were unconscious and that the trainers took you to the training area instead of through the chute. And he was going to allow it."

"See, I told you," Richard said.

"Yeah, well next time you need to remember to collapse at the end of the chute, not at the finish line. Nationals are in Knoxville, Tennessee, and I guarantee you will be DQ'd there. Now let's get our shit together and head up there. They're going to put the final scores on the scoreboard in a few minutes."

Richard grabbed his spike bag and walked up alongside Devlin. "So who won the race?"

"Johnson won by less than a second. It was a great race," Devlin said.

"Wow, I'm sorry I wasn't up there."

"Did you try your hardest?" Devlin asked.

"Well, I threw up and passed out. I doubt I could have gone any faster. Yeah, I guess I tried my hardest."

"Then you have nothin' to be sorry about," he said, and put his arm around Richard. "I'm proud of you, Rickey-boy."

"You think we won?"

"I don't know. We'll see in a few minutes."

When they reached the golfhouse, Richard spotted Susan, who ran up to him and threw her arms around him. He thought to himself, "A hug like this is worth throwing up for."

"You were awesome," she said.

"Well, we'll see how awesome in a few minutes," he said.

"What? You don't know what place you got?"

"No. I know I finished fourth. But we don't have team scores yet. Devlin says it's because I knocked out the scoring computer when I collapsed at the finish line."

Susan started laughing when she heard that. "That's great. You are so hard core," she said and planted a soft kiss on his lips and even slipped him the tongue. Richard was a little apprehensive about swapping spit since he'd thrown up. But she didn't seem to mind, so neither did he.

Phil and Atlas came up and congratulated him. Richard told them that their congrats were a bit premature since the team scores weren't out and his individual performance meant nothing without knowing how the team did.

Nearly 1,000 people were packed in the small area around the scorer's table and underneath the scoreboard. Fans, athletes, coaches and some officials all stood there talking to the person next to them, all the while keeping an eye on the scoreboard to see if the team scores would flash and end the mystery.

Finally something did come up—scores for the women's race. That race was no mystery. Georgia, the defending NCAA women's champions, won the meet easily—placing five runners in the top ten. The scoreboard then flashed the women's individual results. This made sense since the women's race went off first, but Richard was impatient and wanted the great mystery to end.

Then the scoreboard flashed in big yellow letters, "MEN'S TEAM RESULTS". It seemed to flash those same three words for about 10 minutes just to tantalize everyone. But then the results came up and the top three lines read like this:

1. F.I.T. —50 (4,5,6,16,19)

2. Tennessee—51 (1,10,11,14,15)

3. Kentucky—53 (3,8,12,13,17)

The crowd, mostly Aggie supporters, screamed and celebrated. Susan threw her arms around Richard, who had his arms up in the air and had a look of disbelief on his face. Anthony and Jeff grabbed Richard and dragged him to the ground where the rest of the team piled on. Devlin brought out champagne and gave every member of the team a bottle as they got off the pile.

Richard couldn't drink champagne. He drank almost three bottles in one night at his own New Year's Eve party during his senior year in high school. He threw up for two days afterward. The taste of champagne made him ill ever since. But he gladly took the bottle, shook it up, popped the cork, and sprayed Anthony, Jeff and everyone else within a five-yard vicinity.

Johnny and Hargrove came up from behind Richard and tackled him.

"You better be ready to party tonight," Johnny said as they wrestled on the ground.

"Just tell me where it is and I'm there," said Richard. As the three sat on the ground, they contemplated the best site for the party, and decided on the Clubhouse. Richard went up to Susan, Phil and Atlas, who were watching Richard get tackled over and over by different people. Richard was covered head to toe in dirt and looked like a 10-year-old who'd just been caught tearing up his mother's garden.

"Are you all right?" Susan asked jokingly.

"I'll recover," he smiled. "So it looks like I'm throwing the party. Are you guys down with it?" he asked Phil and Atlas. They nodded in the affirmative. "I figured you would be," Richard said to them. "And what about you?" he asked Susan, almost positive what the answer would be.

"I don't know, dude," she said. "I think you need to party with the boys tonight."

"I'd like to party with everyone," he responded quickly.

"I don't think so. I don't think I'm in the mood for the kind of partying you guys are gonna do tonight."

"You mean you're not in the mood for a beer-guzzling pukefest? What a shock!" he said sarcastically.

She started laughing along with Phil and Atlas. He didn't join in their laughter, though. She saw that his comment was serious and apologized. But Richard wanted none of it.

"No, don't apologize," he said. "I'm gonna have a good time tonight with or without you."

"You'll probably have a better time without me," she said, trying to make him feel better about her absence. That didn't work, either.

"No, I won't have a better time," he said. "Just as I wouldn't have a better time if Phil and Atlas weren't there. When something good happens to me, I like to celebrate with my friends. And I know that you could be there if you wanted to, but you just don't fucking feel like it. And that's what really hurts."

Richard saw out of the corner of his eye that Phil and Atlas were looking at the ground and were embarrassed about being present at this argument. He didn't care, though. He wanted Susan to feel guilty about not coming to the party, and he seemed to be doing a good job.

"I just wish you'd tell me it's because you don't want people to think we're going out. Because it sure as hell ain't that you want to give me my space and allow me time with 'The Boys.'"

"Come on, Richard. You're reading way too much into this thing," she said.

"I'm sure I am," he said, and then looked at Phil and Atlas. "I'll see you guys tonight. Naked kegstands all around."

Phil and Atlas laughed and Richard turned around and left. Susan called to him, but he just ignored her. He knew he'd make up with her the next day. He just didn't want to deal with it right then. He caught up with Johnny and Hargrove and hopped in the flatbed of Hargrove's truck. He opened the window to the front cab and said, "Where to boys?"

"We need to go back to the trailer and drink some shots before we do anything," said Hargrove, who was clearly in command of the activities for the rest of the day.

As Hargrove backed out of his parking spot, Richard spotted his three roommates and motioned for them to come along and join in the festivities. Hargrove waited while the three sprinted to the truck and jumped in. Mad Dog let out a howl and the truck sped away.

5

Hargrove's Philosophy

The season was over. Richard had completed the first part of his mission. Two weeks after the SEC's, he led his team to a first place finish at the NCAA Region III Championships at Furman, South Carolina, which includes every school south of Virginia. He placed fourth behind the same trio of Johnson, Allen and Bird. Mad Dog placed sixth, and Williams was ninth.

Once again, the surprise of the meet for Richard was the walk-on Bache, who placed 32nd as the Aggies' fourth man. Jeff was the team's fifth man in 35th place. Bache's performance, just like the conference meet, won the day for the Aggies—a narrow three-point victory over Tennessee.

Richard and the Aggies did it again ten days later at the NCAA Championships in Knoxville, Tennessee—home of the Vols.

In that race, Richard went out in his typically cautious style, and started passing runners after the mile mark. He never stopped passing runners throughout the race. Over the last quarter-mile he kicked by five runners to finish fifth. One runner he passed on the homestretch was the Olympic 1500-meter champ, a Kenyan, who was competing for Mount St. Mary's College. Another athlete he blew by on the homestretch was "The Shadow," Jim Bird.

The day before the race, Richard strutting like a professional wrestler, told Bird, "You're going down." Bird playfully responded by saying, "You can forget about all that SEC brotherhood crap. You're on your own tomorrow." Bird finished seventh and bought Richard's first beer after the race.

The race came down to a sprint and a Kenyan running for Iowa State, got the better of Tennessee's Johnson and Arkansas's Allen. Arkansas won the team title. The Kenyans combined to put Iowa State in second place. But the big surprise was the third place finish of the unheralded Aggies from FIT, who beat the fourth place Volunteers by a mere five points. Along with

Richard's fifth place finish, Mad Dog finished 19th and Williams finished 23rd. Jeff came in 65th, and Dante was the team's fifth man in 97th, while Gopher finished in 154th. The freshman Bache went out with the leaders and fell apart. He came in 172nd, tenth from last.

Devlin had given the distance runners a week off from practice to rest and study for final exams, which were a week away, in the second week of December. The time off from practice was nice, but it didn't translate into a complete vacation. Devlin still had the team running 40 miles that week. But compared to the mileage, workouts, and races they'd been through, 40 miles was a walk in the park. Richard took the time to revel in his recent glory and blow off some steam. So there he was on a cool early December afternoon, drinking beers at the Windjammer with Johnny and Hargrove.

As usual, Richard was being careful about his drinking. He made sure that he drank only one glass of beer per pitcher. But he was sitting with two lifetime alcoholics and after a couple of hours, they'd put down six pitchers. Richard was feeling tipsy after his six beers. Hargrove and Johnny, who'd had about 12 or 13 each, were hammered.

After a great season, an athlete will often get a feeling of invincibility. The solid buzz in Richard's head from the alcohol only enhanced that feeling, which he'd been experiencing since he crossed the finish line at NCAAs. "You know fellas, sometimes I think about giving up the whole damn sport," Richard said, looking down the bar at his compatriots. "But then something happens, like last week, and I say, I'm gonna stick with competitive running until I'm 35."

"No, you won't," Hargrove said matter of factly, looking down at his beer mug.

"What?" Richard said with a confused look on his face.

"I said, no you won't," Hargrove said with emphasis, staring straight at Richard. "You'll be lucky if you're running at 35. And it certainly won't be competitive running on any serious level. It'll be jogging 40 miles a week at seven-minute pace."

"I can be competitive 13 years down the road, Hargrove. My body was meant for running. I don't get injured."

Hargrove and Johnny laughed out loud when he said that. Richard took offense.

"It's true, I've never had any kind of injury that's kept me from running," he said in almost a cocky tone.

"Let me tell you something, Dick," Hargrove said as he sat up. All of a sudden, he looked serious and sober . "The most efficient human body in the world was not meant to withstand the training it takes to be good. You know that every time you go over a hurdle in the steeplechase you do a little more damage to your back?" Hargrove said. "I've seen you stretch at practice, and already I see the signs of a degenerative back problem."

"Well, that's why I'm quitting the steeple after the Olympic Trials," Richard retorted.

"So what are you gonna do?" Hargrove asked. "5K-10K?"

Richard nodded defensively.

"Give me a break, Dick," Hargrove said, sounding annoyed. "First of all, I want to make sure we're talking about the same thing. You're talking about making a few grand from road races in the fall and winter and then hitting the track in the spring to make the Olympic team. Right?" Richard nodded yes. "Good. Because after college, if you're going to train seriously and your goal isn't to make money and make the Olympic team, then you're wasting your time. You might as well just get a full-time job and run five miles a day like every other jolly-jogger out there."

Richard realized he'd touched a nerve in Hargrove, who hadn't picked up his beer glass since he started talking. Richard didn't want to see Hargrove work himself into a lather, but he did want to stick around to hear his point.

"Now, if you're thinking 5K-10K, you're really thinking 10K," Hargrove continued. "Because your real event is always the longer of the two that you're thinking about running. If you were serious about the 5K you'd have said 'Mile-5K' instead of '5K-10K.' So it's the 10K. Now, if you want to make the Olympic team in the 10K there're only two ways to do it. One way is to run 70 miles a week and do hellacious track workouts. But you have to have the speed and strength of a world class miler, which you most definitely do not possess, Dick. You may be able to outkick a bunch of college kids in the SEC and run a 4:02 mile indoor. But the boys in the big time would have you for lunch in a mile or a 5K. The other way is to hammer at least 100 miles per week, which is what most of the big timers do, even if they are great milers.

"It doesn't matter how you do it, though, because either way the training is going to kill you. If it's not the 100 miles week after week, it's all those intervals on the track in your spikes."

"I think I can handle it," Richard said. This angered Hargrove even more.

"You think you can?" he said. He was getting louder. "Dick, you don't know shit! What kind of mileage did you do this fall, 75 per week?" Richard nodded. "Try adding 25 miles a week to your training, plus two tough workouts a week. Trust me, Dick. I never got injured before I started training at that level, and then I fell apart like a house of cards."

Richard cut in. "I think your finish had less to do with your knee, Hargrove, and more to do with this," he said pointing at Hargrove's beer mug, which he still hadn't lifted since their conversation began. Richard was sorry he said what he did, but the New Yorker in him wouldn't let Hargrove get away so easily. Hargrove was steamed, but he maintained his composure.

"Let me tell you what happens when you start running 100 miles per week, every week," Hargrove said in a quiet, intense voice that Richard had never heard before. "It takes a couple of months to get used to the mileage, but after that you feel pretty good for a while. You get some aches and pains which you, of course, run through and ignore. Then after a while the pain becomes too great to ignore, so you start popping the Advil or some other anti-inflammatory that the doctor gives you. But you keep on running through it, ignoring the signs your body's giving you to take some time off. Pretty soon the pain is so great that you can't run, even though you've popped so many Advils that you're shitting blood. You go to the doctor and he tells you it's a knee, an ankle, a stress fracture, a ruptured disk, a degenerative hip, a sciatic nerve, or something else that's going to require surgery and/or therapy and your immediate retirement from competitive running.

"It may take six months. It may take six years. But it will happen sooner or later, Dick. No distance runner ever *decides* to retire. Distance runners are *forced* into retirement by Mother Nature and Father Time. No one retires from this sport unscathed. You leave this sport in some state of pain. Either it's the physical pain of training too hard to get to the top, or it's the mental pain of never getting there. Sometimes it's both.

"And don't go thinking that you're an exception to the rule. Because there are no exceptions to this rule. You can only train beyond your limits for a certain amount of time before your body calls it quits. Name me a great American distance runner and I'll name you the injury that forced him into retirement. You gonna tell me that your body was more meant for running than Mary Decker? Shit, I need all my fingers and toes to count the number of times she's been under the knife. What about Shorter, Liquori, and Ryun? All of them ended their careers in pain. If Prefontaine hadn't died in that car crash at 24, he would have trained himself into retirement as well."

"What about the ones that are still world class at 38?" Richard asked.

"They didn't start training seriously till they were 33," Hargrove responded quietly. "That's why they're world class that late in life.

"I'm not trying to tell you this stuff to put you down, Dick," Hargrove softened. "You're a damn good runner. But it's important that you understand now that great distance runners aren't like great basketball players. They don't go down in a blaze of glory and ride off into the sunset with the girl and a few million in the bank. Distance runners retire quietly and roll off into the dark night in their wheelchairs with little or nothing financially to show for their efforts. For all but a few of us, this is a 'born to lose, live to win' sport. I just don't want to see you get out of college and get your hopes up over something that isn't there. I've seen too many guys like you jump onto the road race circuit all excited, expecting to race every weekend and make thousands of dollars. The roads take a lot out of you physically. And you're in trouble if you line up at the start saying, 'If I don't win, I can't pay rent.' Come February, when all the big money races are in this state, every African you've ever heard of, and many more that you haven't, are gonna be here trying to do the same thing you are—get rich on the roads. And believe me, they're prepared to do it."

With that, Hargrove shut up, picked up his beer mug and deposited the half-glass remaining down his gullet. He filled his mug again and quickly downed that, almost in an effort to make up for all the drinking time lost while talking. Nothing was said for a while, as Richard took in what Hargrove had said. Hargrove was someone who rarely wanted to be taken seriously. But Richard knew deep down that Hargrove was right in what he'd said. Still, though, it was Hargrove talking.

"Born to lose, live to win!" Richard finally said. "Where

the hell did you come up with that one?" Hargrove started to laugh and sprayed beer out of his mouth onto Richard, which made Johnny and Richard laugh hysterically along with him.

The threesome parted ways about 5 p.m. When Richard got home, he walked in the door and was attacked by the aroma that was Mad Dog and Gin. Gin had spent every night—and almost every day—at The Clubhouse since her arrival at Dick Stomp. She was a mild annoyance to Richard at first, but now she was beginning to make him lose sleep over the issue of her extended stay.

He would have had no problem telling her to haul ass in the first week if she slept on the couch. But because she slept upstairs in Mad Dog and Gopher's room, he felt it wasn't his place to say anything. It was Gopher's place. And since Gopher was even more afraid of confrontation than he was afraid of Gin, he didn't say anything and just began sleeping on the couch.

Jeff was similar to Gopher in that respect, always preferring to stay neutral in an argument. Richard had nicknamed Jeff "Switzerland" because of that character trait. Jeff, who also felt it was Gopher's job to get rid of her, wasn't afraid to live in filth either. But even he was beginning to get tired of the "fragrance."

Richard, on the other hand, was not afraid of confrontation or Gin. He was getting to the point where any day, he was going to tell them both to shape up or get out. He walked in the living room and saw Gopher sitting there on the puke couch. Newspapers, plates of food, cups, clothes and pizza boxes covered up most of the room's brown carpet.

"Excuse me," he said to Gopher. "Did a tornado touch down in this room?"

Gopher laughed at the question. "Yeah, this place is a shithole," he said and gave the room a look around as well. "God, this place is disgusting," he said with an air of frustration.

"You know, Gopher. Our problems have a name," he said referring obviously to Gin.

"They are so gross," Gopher agreed. "You should see our room. I don't even sleep up there any more because it's so awful."

"I know. So why don't you exercise your right as a rent

payer and kick her out? And while you're at it, have her take the Mad Dog with her."

"Yeah, I need to do something. I'm getting tired of sleeping on the couch," Gopher said. "But I'm no good at these things. Why don't you do it?"

"Me? Damn it, Gopher. Could you not be a wimp for about two minutes and go upstairs and lay down the law?"

"I can't," he said weakly.

"You make me sick," he paused and thought about going upstairs and kicking them out himself, but decided against it.

"No, I'm not gonna say anything. This is your job. I'll back you up, and I'm sure Jeff will too. But this is all you, Gopher. When you decide you're tired of sleeping on the couch, let me know," he said and walked into his room, his one place of refuge left in the whole apartment.

"I'm tired of it now," Gopher shouted to him.

"Not tired enough," Richard responded from his room.

Winter Break

The winter break came and all the residents of The Clubhouse went home for the holidays except Richard.

For Richard, going home always involved distractions. There were his friends, who were always convincing him to stay out till all hours of the morning. There were family functions with his grandparents and cousins that would be organized just because he was home for a few weeks. And then there was the cold—one of the main reasons he went to FIT in the first place.

When Richard was in high school, there were many days that he would bundle up for a run, step outside, feel that cold wind blow right through him, turn around, go back inside, and call it a day.

The night before he left for his recruiting trip to FIT, he'd gone on a midnight run. It was late November and unseasonably cold. He froze his butt off on that run. When he got down to Arboretum, it was seasonally warm. He was sold. He realized a few years later that that one midnight run had a disproportionate influence in his decision of where to attend college.

He had a somewhat different attitude toward the weather now than he had when he was in high school. If he could run while he was home, he would run, no matter what the temperature. But there would be many days when he couldn't run because the roads were too icy and the grass was covered knee-high with snow. And there would be no days where it would be warm enough to run an interval track workout.

The indoor track season went by fast, and if he went home he would not be ready for prime time when he came back. He wanted to concentrate on his training during the break, without the distractions of social engagements and the weather. He wanted to be ready for Arkansas and Tennessee when they came to Arboretum in late February for the SEC Indoor Championships. Therefore, he needed to stay in Arboretum for winter break.

Since he couldn't go to New York, his parents came down to Arboretum for a week. They left on a Friday morning, stayed overnight in a motel in South Carolina, and arrived in Arboretum Saturday afternoon.

They'd planned to stay in a motel while in Arboretum, but Richard told them not to bother. No one was at his apartment, so he had plenty of beds.

"Is it habitable, Richard?" his mother asked over the phone.

"Oh sure, Mom, you'll love it," he said while surveying the living room, which looked like Hurricane Central.

Richard spent the entire Friday before their arrival cleaning up: dishes, floors, carpets, bedrooms, living room, bathrooms. He even removed the cushions from the puke couch, unzipped the covers, and washed them. At the end of the day, the only part of the house that would be recognizable to his roommates were the walls, which were finger-painted at Dick Stomp.

He thought about pinning something up to cover some of the racier inscriptions on the wall, but he decided against it. His parents were a part of the Woodstock generation; they were stuck in the traffic the concert created on the New York Thruway, and almost gave birth prematurely to Richard. He figured they could handle some raunchy comments on the wall.

When his parents showed up, they told him that Evan, his 13-year-old brother, had to stay in New York at a friend's house because he had varsity wrestling tournaments over the break. Richard was disappointed that he wouldn't get to see his brother, but he understood the situation. After all, he was do-ing the same thing by staying in Arboretum.

Richard sat on the recently-cleaned puke couch and got all the dirt on his little brother. His parents told him that little Evan, who was now in 8th grade, was a starter on the varsity wres-tling team in the 125 lb. weight-class. He weighed only five pounds less than Richard.

They sat there and reminisced. Richard could remember when he was in high school and Evan, who was seven or eight years old, would come home from the elementary school wres-tling clinic and practice the moves he'd learned that day on Richard. Their father would sit in a chair off to the side and watch with a big smile on his face as Richard would dutifully take his licks as Evan demonstrated what he'd learned. Evan took great joy in doling out sanctioned punishment to his older brother.

Occasionally, Evan would get a little overzealous and throw Richard down on the carpet a little too hard. When that hap-pened, Richard would make him pay by resisting on the next move, making it difficult for Evan to complete the fall. Evan would get frustrated and start doing anything he could think of to get his older brother down. Richard would then use his superior strength to take Evan down and pin him—just to show him who was boss.

Evan didn't like to lose—his competitive desire might have been even greater than Richard's—and he'd get red in the face with anger when Richard held him down. The longer Richard held him down, the redder Evan's face became, until Richard decided he'd had enough. He'd hop off and roll into a ball to protect himself because Evan would be swinging as soon as his arms were free. Richard loved the feisty character his brother had.

Evan was tough and he only weighed 80 lbs. back then. He was 125 lbs. now. Although Richard was strong for his 130-lb. weight, he imagined that his brother could probably take him on the wrestling mat now.

"Imagine how tough that kid's gonna be when he's a se-nior," he told his parents. "I feel sorry for his competitors."

"The hell with them," his father said, "I feel sorry for the guy who'll be matched up with him in practice every day. They'll have to give that kid a Congressional Medal of Honor if he makes it through the season."

"Or a Purple Heart if he doesn't," Richard chimed in.

Susan came over later in the evening and met the parental units. Mom had trouble believing she was older than 25, let alone 32.

The three Dubins spent Sunday doing exactly what they would be doing if they were in New York. Richard and his father watched pro football and tossed the football outside. His mother went shopping and cooked about a week's worth of food. She also sat in on a few football plays. Unlike many women her age, she understood the game and knew what was going on. She just wasn't as big a fan as her husband and older son.

On Monday, Richard took his parents up to Devlin's office. After his parents and Devlin exchanged pleasantries, they excused themselves. Richard had told them on their way up to the office that he had business to discuss in private with Devlin. His parents understood and agreed to hang around the football stadium until he was done.

When they walked out and shut the door, Devlin turned to Richard and said, "How's it goin', Rickey-boy?"

"Good. Let's talk about my mission for this upcoming season." he said abruptly, sidestepping the small talk. He knew Devlin wouldn't mind.

"Rickey-boy, your mission is to win an SEC title this season."

"That's pretty vague," Richard said. "What event?"

"I don't know yet," Devlin said. "Could be mile, 3K, or 5K. We'll have to see how your training's going."

"What about the team?"

"Rickey, you're our leader. And I kinda feel like I did in cross country, that you set an example to every sprinter, jumper, thrower and distance runner when you run. But track is different than cross country. Only five on a team score in cross. We've had 25 score in track at the conference meet before—and we lost that one."

"I remember. I was there," Richard said bitterly, referring to the outdoor championships his freshman year when FIT finished a close second to Louisiana State.

"Arkansas and Tennessee are tough," Devlin said, stating the obvious. "You'll have your hands full with their distance crew. You don't need to worry about what the rest of the team is doing. If you get it done in your events, I have a feeling we'll get it done as a team."

"What about nationals?"

"I ain't worried about nationals," Devlin said. "If you have a good conference meet, you'll finish top two or three in some event at the NCAAs."

"So that's it for indoor? One conference title and a top three finish at nationals? Would you like mustard or relish with that, sir?"

They laughed and then talked about his workouts for the next few weeks. Devlin agreed to meet him at the track on Tuesdays and Fridays over the next two weeks to supervise, add moral support—and comic relief—and to time his intervals. Richard mentioned that his parents wanted him to go down to Miami later in the week for a few days to visit family.

"Jesus Christ, Rickey boy. It's Christmas. Of course you can go see your family," Devlin said, forgetting the fact that Richard's family didn't celebrate Christmas. "I personally think it'd be a great idea as long as you think it won't be stressful to you and it'll take your mind off your mission for a while."

"Well, I'm gonna run while I'm down there. I won't slack off. And I'll be back for Friday's workout," Richard said almost apologetically.

"That's fine. But you're not getting what I'm saying, Rickey boy. You need to settle down a little. The indoor conference meet's not for two months. You're gonna give yourself a nervous breakdown if you don't take a little bit of a mental breather. I tell you what. Let's call off Friday's workout so you can spend an extra couple of days with your family. All right?"

"You sure?"

"One workout in December ain't gonna make the difference," Devlin said. "We'll workout tomorrow and then I'll see you next week. Take some time with your family. And for Chrisake, try to quit thinking about the other teams so much. You're gonna kick their butts."

They parted ways and Richard told his parents about the extra time he had on his hands. They spent the rest of the day walking around the virtually uninhabited FIT campus and stayed in Miami from Tuesday night until Sunday. Richard's parents rested up on Monday and left Arboretum Tuesday morning, leaving Richard to his lonesome until classes started the following Monday.

Gopher and Jeff came back from vacation the day before classes started. While surfing the Atlantic at his parents' house in Melbourne, Gopher decided he'd had enough of Devlin, the team, and the sport in general. Richard knew what that meant: a semester of guiltless drinking, hellraising, and laying around the house watching MTV. Richard found him pathetic, although he could admit to being slightly jealous.

Jeff spent his time shoveling snow and drinking beer with his and Richard's high school buddies. While Jeff gave Richard the update on everyone back home, he announced his retirement from the sport, as well. Jeff's reasons were more noble than Gopher's, though. Jeff was a senior, and he needed to start looking for a job before he graduated. Unlike Gopher, Jeff's parents couldn't afford to pay for college. Jeff had $20,000 in loans that he would have to start paying as soon as they handed him his degree. At the same time, though, it was Jeff's last semester in college and he wanted to make it a memorable one
.   Richard could excuse Jeff from wanting one four-month period of guilt-free partying before entering "the real world." For Gopher, though, Richard had lost all respect.

It was going to be a trying semester for Richard, who was beginning to feel alone and isolated in his pursuit of the mission. Not having his two roommates hurting alongside him only intensified those feelings.

Eviction

It was a week after classes started in Richard's tenth semester at FIT. The Clubhouse was up to its usual routine. Richard and Jeff were in their respective rooms, working on separate projects for the same class. They were both journalism majors and political science minors.

Gopher was in the new Lazy Boy chair watching T.V. They found the new chair next to a nearby dumpster a few days earlier. They decided it must have been a Christmas gift from the Tahiti Apartments management for being such good tenants.

Mad Dog and Gin were wrestling on the puke couch. A white bedsheet was the only piece of cloth that kept them from complete nudity. Richard, who was studying with his door open, could hear their laughing and giggling as they rolled around on the couch and floor. It annoyed him, but he was not motivated to say anything. Gopher was motivated.

In a completely uncharacteristic display, Gopher got up from the Lazy Boy and shouted, "Why don't you shut up and put some clothes on, you fucking morons! I'm sick of looking at your naked asses all the time."

Out from the huge lump underneath the sheet came Gin's head, which said, "Fuck you, Gopher."

"NO!" came a scream from Richard's room. He'd heard it all and finally snapped. He threw down the book he was reading. He rushed into the living room and screamed at Gin, "Fuck you, you non-rent paying bitch!

"I pay rent here," Richard continued "and I am sick and tired of you, your boyfriend, and the shithole you've made of this place. You have no respect for this place, the people who live here, or yourselves. You've made this place a disgusting, depressing place to live and I can't take it anymore.

"I'm gonna do what I should have done at the start," he said. "I'm giving the both of you one week to find a place. If you ain't out by then, I'm throwing your stuff into the yard."

Richard started to walk away but feared they wouldn't take him seriously. He turned back around and said, "One more thing. Don't either of you try and fuck with me on your way out. I haven't hit a girl since sixth grade, but if you fuck with me, Gin, I ain't afraid to break your fucking face. Your dentist and plastic surgeon will be able to retire after they get done with you."

He turned and as he was walking away he said once more for emphasis, "ONE WEEK!"

Richard didn't see Mad Dog and Gin around the apartment after his tirade. They found a place in another apartment complex on 34th Street—about a mile from Tahiti Apartments—and had all their stuff removed less than a week later.

Mad Dog wouldn't talk to Richard for a few weeks afterward. But for Richard, it was small price to pay for his sanity.

The Wedding

One week after he booted Mad Dog and Gin out of the Clubhouse, Richard came home from practice to hear the news.

"Hey, Dick. What are you doing tomorrow afternoon?" Gopher asked.

"Nothing besides practice," he said. "What's going on?"

"Mad Dog and Gin are getting married."

"You're kidding."

"Don't you want to know where it's going to be?" Gopher asked, itching to impart the information.

"Why? I'm sure I'm not invited after what occurred last week."

"Hell, Mad Dog doesn't give a shit anymore," Gopher said. "You know him, he can't hold a grudge. Besides, he was more than happy to get out of this place."

"Then why hasn't he talked to me in a week?"

"How often did he talk to you before? He's not the most talkative person in the world, Dick."

"That's true. Do you think he wants me to be there?"

"Yeah. He wants everyone in town there."

"What about Gin?"

"She's the same way. She just wants it to be a big party."

"All right, I'll bite. Where's it going to be?" Jeff came down the steps and foiled Gopher by giving the news first. "Tomorrow. 5 p.m. Charlie's Pizza Palace buffet counter. Be there!"

"What are you talking about, Jeff?" said Richard, who was confused.

"They're getting married at Charlie's tomorrow," said Gopher, who was downright giddy at the prospect of such weirdness.

"Why?" Richard asked.

"Because they're fucking nuts," Jeff said.

"Of course, how silly of me," Richard said. "You know, every once in a while I start to think that behind all the madness, those two may actually have a drop of sane blood in them. And then they do something like this and prove me dead wrong. . . Any guess as to what they're gonna wear?"

"I don't know," Gopher said. "But I guarantee tomorrow is going to be an experience. I'm so excited, I'm going to have to get drunk just to fall asleep tonight."

The next day, Devlin called Richard early in the morning and demanded that he come up to the athletic office immediately. Richard got out of bed, brushed his teeth and pedaled up to campus, over an hour before his 10 a.m. class. He was nervous because Devlin sounded serious. He wasn't sure what he'd done wrong or who he'd pissed off, but he was already in the defensive mode when he walked into Devlin's office.

"What's the problem now, Devlin?"

"What the fuck is goin' on in that apartment you live in?" Devlin said.

"Get to the point, please."

"I hear that stupid roommate of yours, Ledbetter, is gonna marry Crazy Gin today. What the fuck is goin' on?"

Richard paused for a moment in shock. The news had been out less than 24 hours and Devlin knew about it already. Devlin was always great at finding out information. But who was his snitch? Richard didn't want to ask that question because that would let on that he knew more about it than Devlin. The question became: How much did Devlin know? The answer was to play dumb.

"First of all, in case you haven't heard, Mike Ledbetter is not my roommate any more. I kicked him and his girlfriend out last week. They're fucking pigs. I have no idea where they're living," he said, anticipating the question of their whereabouts. "Secondly, I probably know less about this wedding than you, believe it or not. I know it's today, I don't know when or where.

"And by the way, Devlin. You got a lot of nerve waking me up, dragging me down to the office, scaring me to death that I did something wrong, all so you can get some gossip about something that's really not your business in the first place." Richard derived much satisfaction in lashing out at Devlin. But as usual, Devlin had a comeback.

"Listen up, partna. When I have a scholarship athlete who's fuckin' up his life and endangering his scholarship, it's my responsibility to get that kid help. Kinda like I did with you a few years ago. And that sumbitch Mad Dog needs help." He paused to deposit some lip juice into the Coke can on his desk before continuing. "Tell me something, Rickey. How do you think his parents are gonna feel when they find out what's goin' on?"

"I doubt they care."

"The fuck they don't," Devlin snapped back. "I was on the phone with his mother for almost an hour this morning. She was crying for most of our conversation."

Richard was genuinely shocked, although it wasn't beyond Devlin to embellish or flat-out lie to make his point.

"So what are you saying, Devlin? You're gonna stop the wedding?" Surely Devlin wouldn't go to that length, Richard thought. Or would he?

"I don't know," he said. "I wanna talk to him and find out what's goin' on in that fucked-up head of his. Then I want him to call his parents and tell them what's goin' on before anything serious happens."

"Well, good luck on your crusade, Devlin. I admire it. But I think it's a wasted effort."

"Rickey, I want you to tell him to come to my office today."

"I probably won't see him before practice, Devlin. Remember, he lives elsewhere now. But if I do, I'll be sure to tell him you're looking for him," he said.

As he got up to walk out the door he took one more shot at Devlin for good measure. "Do me a favor, Devlin. Next time you want to drag me in the middle of something that's none of my business, would you do it over the phone, and could it wait till after 9 a.m.?"

By practice time the whole team was buzzing. Everyone was coming up to Richard, asking him what exactly was going on.

Richard knew nothing and said so. He'd gone home after class, told Gopher what had been said by Devlin, and went to practice from there.

Looking around, Richard noticed that the assistant coaches were running the practice that afternoon. Devlin, he assumed, must have been on a manhunt.

Practice consisted of an easy eight-miler and some 100-meter strides, which he did barefoot on the grass. When he was done, he biked straight to Charlie's. It was 4:50 p.m. and the wedding was scheduled to start at 5 p.m.

He arrived and saw many of his friends including Jeff, Phil, Atlas and Mary. They were sitting at a table, drinking a pitcher of beer. Richard went up to the counter, ordered a pitcher and a slice, pulled a chair up to their table and began imbibing quickly. He felt he needed at least a buzz to experience the bizarre ceremony.

Richard was more than buzzed at 5:45 p.m. when Gopher ran in. Gopher was sweaty and out of breath when he came into Charlie's—which was now packed with spectators who were expecting something memorable.

"Dudes, you won't believe what's been going on," Gopher started. He took a seat as Phil filled up a cup of beer for him. "Mad Dog and Gin came running into the apartment about an hour ago. Mad Dog says, 'Hide us! Hide us! The Devil's after us.' So I told them to go hide upstairs. Then, not a minute later, Devlin bursts in, comes into the living room and says, 'Where's Mad Dog?' I told him I don't know. All of a sudden you hear these footsteps running down the stairs out back. Devlin hears them and dashes out the back door. Well, those crazy fuckers jump into the pool and hide underwater till the Devil is gone. They were so scared of getting caught they didn't even come up to breathe.

"So when the Devil left, they got out of the pool, and jumped into her Jeep. I guess they wanted to go to their place to get some dry clothes for the wedding. Well, Devlin was waiting for them. He chased them in his car all the way around the parking lot. He finally cornered them by the storage shed in the back of the complex. He got out of the car and dragged Mad Dog back to our place and made him call his parents and tell them what was going on."

"So what'd they say?" Richard asked.

"Mad Dog said they didn't care," Gopher said. "But it was fucking hilarious hearing Devlin yell at him. Mad Dog said his devil eye turned white. Of course, when I heard them coming I ran upstairs to my room. I didn't want to get in the middle of that shit."

"Of course," Richard said sarcastically. Above all, Gopher always avoided conflict. "So when are they getting here? The crowd's getting a bit restless. Well, the ones that are sober anyway."

"They should be here any minute now. . . Then again, the way the past few hours have gone, you never know," Gopher said. He looked around and surveyed Charlie's Pizza Palace. Seeing that the place was packed with over 100 people, most of whom he recognized, he said, "Holy shit! I can't believe there are this many people here to see this."

"Word spreads fast in this town," Phil said.

Just after 6 p.m. the guests of honor showed up. The bride was wearing a ripped sweatshirt, dumpy shorts, and ratty shoes. The groom was wearing a red and blue plaid flannel shirt buttoned up to the neck, tan pants that had an elastic wasteband with a drawstring, and ratty old running shoes that matched hers. Everyone applauded when they walked in.

The happy couple met with the woman—a notary—who would be performing the ceremony. The three walked up to the counter as if they were going to order some food and began the proceedings.

The whole affair took about five minutes from start to finish. The highlight came when Mad Dog said the words: "To be my wife." Hearing Mad Dog say those words—he said them grandly, as if he were reading one of his poems at a party—made everyone crack up.

All those present seemed to think it was a huge joke, including the groom. Only it was legal, legitimate and very real. Richard still wasn't sure that Mad Dog understood that.

After the ceremony was over, the bride and groom popped open a bottle of champagne, filled some plastic cups, and everyone toasted to their happiness, if that's what this was all about.

That night Gin gave Gopher $100 to buy some kegs. Gopher had decided it was his duty as friend and former roommate to hold the party at The Clubhouse. Richard didn't find this out until Gopher came home and asked him for help in carrying the kegs inside. Richard wasn't happy with the news.

"You must be kidding me?" he screamed. "I live here. Why wasn't I told?"

"I thought you knew," Gopher said lamely. "I told everyone at Charlie's."

"Well, you didn't tell me."

"You must have left early."

"This is bullshit," Richard said in frustration. "I have to kick them out myself without help from anyone else. And even then I can't escape them."

Richard looked at Jeff, who was in the kitchen. "Jeff, you wanna help me out here?"

"I don't care one way or the other," Jeff said with his hands up in the air.

"That's right. I forgot. I live with the man who's afraid of his own shadow and Mr. Switzerland," Richard said.

"This is such bullshit," he said again. "You two quit the team and I suffer because of it."

Richard took the phone in his room and called Susan. "Hey, babe," he said. "I need to ask a favor. . . I need to spend the night at your place tonight. . . I'll explain when I get there. I just need to get the fuck out of this shithole right now, before I lose it. . . Thanks, babe. I'll see you in a few minutes."

Richard threw a change of clothes in a bag and walked out without another word to his two roommates.

4

Getting Ready

Richard never felt better than he did during the weeks leading up to the SEC Indoor Championships. His indoor season had gone smoothly. With two miles in 4:04.7 and 4:05.1, a 3000 in 8:04.2, and numerous solid runs on the 4x800 relay, he'd yet to run a bad race. In fact, he and his teammates had the fastest times in all three events going into the conference meet. Yet Richard still felt like the underdog with something to prove going into the meet. That was because of the presence of the Arkansas foreigners who by now were completely recovered from their fall injuries.

Arkansas loomed over Richard's world like a dark cloud. Since the cross country season had ended, the thought of having to face them at the indoor conference meet bothered him. And the closer he got to the 3000m showdown, the more it began to dominate his thoughts.

The thing that made the Razorbacks so tough was their depth. They had three distance runners who were world class; all were finalists at the World Championships the previous summer. And they had others who weren't far behind.

Richard put himself in a class slightly below that of the top three Arkansas guys, and slightly above the others. On a good day, he could beat them all.

On a bad day, though, they could all beat him. Three guys he didn't have to worry about, though, were Johnson, Allen and Bird, the trio that owned him during cross country. They'd almost certainly run the 5000. Mad Dog would have the pleasure of running against them.

Before the foreigners joined the Arkansas squad, Richard was sure that a bad day at the conference meet would mean a third place finish in his event, at worst. He could live with that on a bad day. Now, though, a bad day could conceivably be sixth or seventh place—an unbearable thought.

So going into the indoor season, he decided to set his sights on the conference meet—which would be at home—and his showdown with Arkansas, rather than focus on the NCAA Championships like most runners of his caliber.

So far, he'd run faster than they had throughout the entire season. But he didn't kid himself. He knew they were a sleeping giant who awoke when seriously challenged. He also knew that while his times were the fastest in the conference so far, they had many guys—some he knew of and some he didn't—capable of running faster. It was these thoughts that obsessed him and interrupted his sleep during the months of January and February.

On Friday, seven days before the indoor conference meet, Richard and Devlin decided that one last tough workout was necessary before a week of rest.

The workout consisted of a mile in 4:25, a fast, hard 3/4 mile in about 3:03, and another mile in 4:25. All intervals had four minutes rest in between. It would be tough, but Richard was ready.

Richard did the workout with Mad Dog and Anthony. He *started* with them anyway. They did the mile in 4:25 together. Richard was jogging, trying hard to hold back from running faster. Anthony and Mad Dog made the time as well, but for them it was a bit more of a struggle.

On the three-quarter interval, Richard took off from the start. He went through the first quarter somewhere between 59 and 60 seconds. He wasn't wearing a watch, choosing instead to run on "feel." He only knew his time because Devlin was calling the lap splits.

At the end of the second lap, Devlin called out his time as 2:00. Richard felt smooth and easy. He could run three seconds slower for his last lap and still make the prescribed time. But he chose instead to press on with the pace.

Coming into the home stretch, Richard resisted the temptation pick it up for the final 100 meters. He wanted to run as smooth and even as possible. Devlin showed him his watch after he crossed the line. It read 2:59.76—a personal best in an interval workout where he was not putting out maximum effort.

Richard smiled when he saw the time. "Still got one more mile to run," he said, trying to keep his mind on the task still ahead.

On the third interval, Richard again broke away quickly

from Mad Dog and Anthony—both of whom had run 3:05 for their three-quarter segment. Richard pushed through the first quarter in 61 seconds, the half in 2:03, and the 3/4 in 3:06.

Going into the last lap, Richard now was beginning to feel a bit tired—but only a little. He concentrated on maintaining the pace, not slowing down for most of the lap and picking up the pace for the last 100 meters—usually tough to do at the end of a hard workout.

As Richard came down the homestretch on the last lap of the mile, his arms and legs worked in harmony. Together they did the work without any strain or struggle. He felt like a machine—an 18-wheeler barreling down a highway at 80 miles per hour. Yet he was barely breathing. He could easily go faster if he wanted. "But why run fast now?" he told himself. "Save as much energy as you can for the meet."

When he came across the finish line, Devlin showed him the watch: 4:07.88. Richard smiled and said calmly, "Holy shit. I must be pretty fit."

"I'd say so," said Devlin, who was seemingly more excited about the workout than Richard. "I think we're gonna have to seriously consider the mile-3,000 double next week."

"I don't care," Richard said. "Just put me in the races you want me to run. I'll take it from there."

Richard was more excited than he let on about the workout. His cool-down run ended conveniently at Susan's house. He gave her a big hug and kiss when she unlocked the door. She was totally enthralled, listening to the first workout of the year that Richard was actually enthusiastic about.

After telling the story of the workout in minute detail, Richard went in Susan's bathroom to take a shower. She joined him a few minutes later. They came out of the steamy room 30 minutes later, warm and satisfied. He spent the night there, sleeping soundly for the first time in over a week. For one night, his worries about the upcoming meet were absent from his dreams.

Hell Night

Friday night. Midnight. The night before the meet. Richard

had felt tired three or four hours earlier, but decided to stay awake so that maybe he could fall asleep around 10 or 11 p.m. and get a decent night's rest for a change. Now at midnight, wide awake and realizing his plans for sleep were wishful thinking, he was kicking himself for not taking that nap when he had the chance.

What really irked him, though, was that Susan said she would come over around 11 p.m. He'd been looking forward to her visit all night, especially since the pre-race adrenaline rush kicked in around 10 p.m.

Staring at the TV, Richard felt like an animal, with his apartment as his cage. He needed to see her. He picked up the phone and got her answering machine.

"Susan, this is Richard. I feel like shit and I need to see you. You said you'd come over around 11. I've been waiting for you for over an hour. Please give me a call. It's urgent." He hung up the phone and started breathing heavily.

"She's not around," he said out loud. "How the hell am I going to make it through the night!"

At 1:45 the phone rang. Richard answered it after half a ring.

"Hello," he said, trying to sound calm.

"Hey, babe, how're you doing?" Susan said with a slight slur in her speech.

"Where've you been? You said you'd come over at 11."

"I said I'd come over after I went out with my friends," she said.

"Look, I'm not in the mood to argue about what you said. Just please come over. I need to see you now."

"All right. Relax. I'll be over in a few minutes."

At 2:30 a.m., he heard the engine of her VW Bug pull up and park. He met her at the door with an emotional hug and kiss. He could taste the wine and marijuana on her breath.

He was a bit disappointed. Susan could be tough to get along with when stone-cold sober. He found her even more difficult to deal with when she was high because she would be just as stubborn, but have more trouble keeping her train of thought.

They lay down on his bed and talked for a while. Richard wanted to talk about how he was feeling, but Susan kept veering off topic, spouting random thoughts.

Richard ignored most of her non sequiturs. He was too busy

kissing her neck and grabbing her rump. He was getting hot. But every time he tried to make a major move she rebuffed him, usually by pushing him away just enough so she could roll over.

Once again, their minds were in different universes. Hers was in space, while his was between her legs.

He asked her to sleep over. She said no. He begged her over and over, telling her she was the only thing that could keep him safe and sane through the night. She still said no. He got out of bed in frustration and walked outside.

When he walked out in the parking lot, it occurred to him that he had not ventured outside The Clubhouse since the sun went down, over nine hours earlier. It felt refreshing to be outside, but the relief that came from the change in atmosphere was only temporary. After a few minutes, his nerves and heart rate went sky high again. He measured his pulse at 110 beats per minute—about the rate it beat when he was on a long run.

She came outside soon after. "Babe, what's the matter?" she said.

"You know what's the matter, Susan. It's the night before the biggest and most defining race of my life and I'm dying right now just thinking about the consequences of losing. I can't handle it alone. I need to be with someone."

"I can't help you right now, Richard."

"You've made that abundantly clear."

She came up behind him and put her arms around him. "Look," she said in a quiet, caring voice. "Your race isn't for another 16 hours. I'll come over in the morning and pick you up. We'll spend the day together and I'll help you take your mind off the race. And no matter what happens, we're gonna drink a beer together after this whole thing is over. In the meantime, I want you to get in bed, relax, and think about how much fun we'll have tomorrow. OK?"

He turned around and hugged her tight. "OK," he said. Her short speech had calmed him. He kissed her good night, went inside, crawled into bed, and fell asleep.

The Gardens

Richard awoke at 6 a.m., feeling only somewhat refreshed from his 2^1/$_2$-hour nap. He had only been awake for 30 seconds and the nerves kicked in at high rate. He took his pulse: 115.

He wasn't hungry, but he realized that if he was going to be awake for a long time—which he probably would be on that day—he needed to eat. He went in the kitchen, made two slices of toast with margarine, and ate them in front of the television.

At 7 a.m. he called his parents. He had spoken to them the night before around 9 p.m., before his adrenaline kicked in. Talking to his mother, he told her he actually slept a few hours. Richard could hear his mother relaying the story to his father, who let out a cheer. His dad picked up the phone.

"Congratulations. How'd you do it?"

"Susan came over and calmed me down."

"Great! I like this girl. Are you planning to eat today?" he said sarcastically.

"Yeah," said Richard, who felt too weak to joke. "I had a couple of pieces of toast already. I kind of forced it down, but it stayed down. So that's a moral victory, I suppose."

"Richard, keep in mind you're not in a gulag. You can have more than bread and water today. In fact you *need* more than that to run well," his father said seriously.

"I know. It's just hard to think about food when you have no appetite, Dad."

"I know, son. Just do me a favor. Try and relax and have a good time, tonight. I promise you, your life won't change a great deal if you win or lose. The sun will still rise. You'll still have family and friends that love you. And you'll still have to go to class on Monday."

"I know, Dad. But for me it's a matter of respect. And the only way I can gain it is by winning."

"Jesus, Richard. This is *one* race. Nobody's reputation is made on one race. I mean, how can you enjoy winning if the fear of losing controls your life?"

"I can't," said Richard, who was on the verge of tears listening to his father's painfully true words.

"One of these days, Richard, you've got to learn to take it easier on yourself. Life is not a zero sum game, where you're nothing if you lose. There's more to life than that. I promise you."

"I gotta go," Richard said abruptly. He was losing control of his emotions. He didn't want his father to hear him cry, although he suspected his father knew what was going on.

"OK. Give us a call if you need anything. I love you, son."

"Bye." Richard hung up the phone and put his head down on the kitchen table. The tears flowed.

Richard gathered himself before he called Susan. He didn't want her to know the vulnerable side he showed his parents. He didn't even feel comfortable showing it to them. His emotional release, he had to admit, had done him some good, however. He felt more relaxed than he'd been in weeks.

The phone conversation was quick. He suggested he come over and she agreed. They hung up and he was out the door, making one stop along the way to pick up some orange juice for her hangover.

When he got to her door, she looked like death warmed over. Yet even in her state, she observed that he was considerably more relaxed than the night before. Of course, he couldn't have been any less relaxed, considering the night he'd had. That night he was at the bottom floor emotionally; his elevator could only go up.

When he walked in, he gave her a light hug, knowing she not in the mood for more, considering the way she was feeling. He poured two glasses of orange juice and followed her back to bed. He crawled underneath the warm blanket, gave a big yawn and fell asleep for another half-hour.

He woke up like a shot, and the serenity he'd gained from the talk with his father had run out. He thought that if he called him again he might get a refill. There were no guarantees, though. He didn't want his dad to think he depended on him to get him through a race, although that was truer than Richard wanted to admit.

Suddenly he couldn't sit in bed another second. With a sense of urgency, he got dressed, drank some orange juice, and bugged Susan to get ready so they could leave. He felt trapped indoors and wanted to get out as soon as possible.

They hopped into her Bug and went to Bagelville, the counter-culture bagel joint where hippies were the clientele and ditsy sorority girls the servers. That combination made no sense to Richard. But since most things in Susan's life defied logic, Bagelville made perfect sense. The fact was, she drank their terrible coffee seven days a week, so, that's where the VW Bug automatically went each morning. He wasn't crazy about the place, but he was in no mood to lobby for a change of venue— an argument he would have lost, anyway.

Richard spent a half hour forcing down a cinnamon raisin

bagel with margarine. He tried to read the newspaper while eating, to help take his mind off the race—at least temporarily. It didn't work, though. Instead, he sat in his chair, stared at the grayness of the sports page and felt sorry for himself and the living hell he was putting himself through. He put his hand to his wrist and looked at his watch. His pulse rate was 120.

While Susan took off to do her daily four-mile run, Richard sat in Bagelville and wallowed in his own self-pity until she came back—not that she was helping any.

After she came back, toweled off and stretched thoroughly—the whole process took over an hour, which seemed like an eternity to Richard— the two got into the car.

"Where are we going now?" Richard asked.

Susan responded in her sexy tone. "Just be patient," she said, and planted a soft kiss on Richard's lips.

Richard's normal response to this would have been one of total body excitement. He would have reciprocated her kiss for sure and probably fondled a breast, as well. On that day, though, he felt completely impotent. His sex drive was like a faucet that had been shut too tightly to be turned by a human hand. If anyone had a wrench to loosen him up, it was Susan Connor, but she certainly had her work cut out for her today. Richard was a tough nut to crack the day of a race.

Susan took a right onto University Avenue. Richard shivered as they passed the Dome—the facility that served as the home for FIT's basketball, swimming, gymnastics, and volleyball teams. The Dome also had a 200-meter indoor track and happened to be the site of this year's SEC Indoor Track and Field Championships.

Richard could see the buses that carried all the visiting track teams to this site. Each bus was painted in the colors of the school it represented. He spotted the Arkansas bus. He quickly looked away and began to breathe heavily. Susan saw what he was doing and couldn't resist laughing out loud.

"It's not funny!" Richard said like a hurt child. Susan reached over, kissed his ear and whispered,

"You're gonna kick ass tonight. I'm getting off just thinking about it."

Her words elicited little response from Richard. Susan stayed on University Avenue, taking the road past the Oaks Mall and out of town. In Richard's five years in Arboretum, he had never been this far down the town's main drag.

There was nothing on either side of the road. No stores. No buildings. No houses. No campus. No track. No expectations. No pressures. And the farther they drove, the farther away it all seemed to him. He fantasized that they were just going to keep on driving in whatever direction they were going (he was pretty sure they were headed west). They wouldn't stop except to get gas and food. He dreamed they were leaving behind their lives as they knew them, and starting new ones in another state, with only the clothes on their backs and a few bucks for food. They could both get menial jobs, live in a trailer, and live happily ever after in complete anonymity. It could work. All Susan had to do was keep driving.

After about a half hour of driving on University Avenue, which had changed names about three times since they left town, Susan made a right turn onto a dirt road that was heavily wooded on both sides. She drove another mile until they got to a sign that said "Kanapaha Gardens." She made another right turn into a dirt parking lot. She parked and said, "We're here."

"Where are we?" he asked as they got out of the car.

She took a deep breath and said, "Heaven."

As the two started walking along the trails of Kanapaha, breathing the clean air and taking in the lush foliage, Richard became apprehensive about doing too much walking when he had a race to run in about six hours. Susan allayed his fears, though.

"You have some nervous energy you need to get rid of before you race," she told him. "Now, would you rather just stew in front of a TV set by yourself, thinking about nothing but the race all day long? Or would you rather take a little nature walk with me and think about more pleasant things than those bad-ass runners you're going to beat tonight?"

He couldn't deny her logic, and he went along willingly.

With Susan holding his hand and leading every step of the way, Richard felt completely relaxed and at ease with himself and the surroundings almost immediately. He realized this and uttered a reluctant "Thank you." She smiled and gave him a soft kiss.

After about a half-hour of walking on the trail, Susan took a sudden right turn off the beaten path into the woods. Richard asked, "Where to, now?" But he got no response. She was clearly on a mission of her own and too focused to worry about a question that would be answered soon enough. Richard let the question die in the air and decided to just follow along and wait to find out.

Susan stopped about 100 yards into the woods. She turned around and asked him how he was feeling. Richard gave the shoulder shrug that said he was doing fine.

Susan got down on her knees and Richard followed suit, not really sure what she had in mind. She planted a kiss on his lips, and then another, and then another—each kiss softer and more sensual than the one before.

Richard wasn't sure what Susan was getting at. She often would start things with Richard that she didn't want to finish, so he wasn't sure how far she wanted to take it that day. He found it hard to believe that she, who had refused him so many times in the privacy of her own bedroom, would want to actually get it on in the forest. Then again, he had learned to expect the unexpected from Susan. He also wasn't sure he even wanted to have sex at that moment. In all his self-pity earlier in the day, sex had been the furthest thing from his mind. He was quite sure he was temporarily impotent—a notion that didn't even faze him. But despite the feelings of impotence going through his head, the stirring between his legs was telling him something completely different.

Susan directed Richard to lay on his back. She unzipped him and put her hands between his legs; any fear of temporary impotence was instantly dispelled. Her smile opened wide when she realized that he was all there. She pulled down her pants and began riding him.

Whenever Richard made love to Susan, the thoughts that dominated his mind were of how good it felt to be inside her, and how much he truly loved her. But as he stared up at the cloudless blue sky through a thick layer of leafless branches, he couldn't entirely remove the race from his head.

This is weird, he thought. In a few hours I have to run the SEC championship 3000. But right now I'm in a forest getting it on with this incredible woman. Life is so strange.

Most times they had sex, Richard could outlast Susan. It was, therefore, a shock when Richard reached orgasm after only a few minutes. When she realized what had happened, Susan started laughing. Richard laughed out loud too and they snuggled tightly together.

The two walked out of the forest and back onto the path, hand in hand. Richard had never felt so much love for a person. There was no way, he thought, he could ever love someone as deeply as he loved Susan Connor.

Back To Reality

The VW Bug pulled up to Susan's place at 4 p.m. It was important for Richard to eat about four hours before a race, so on their way back from Kanapaha, they stopped at a fast food joint along University Avenue that featured a pasta bar as well as the stuff behind the counter that Susan referred to as "corporate death burgers."

The pasta bar was just the right call. Richard had some rotelle with plain tomato sauce and a salad that consisted of lettuce, carrots, croutons and a light Italian dressing. He usually liked to put a lot more on a salad, but he didn't want his stomach to have trouble digesting anything heavy or gaseous over the next few hours.

He didn't eat a lot because his body was in race mode. But he ate a plate full of good food that hit the spot. As he walked up the stairs to Susan's apartment, he patted himself on the back for eating the perfect pre-race food, and just the right amount. Eating before a race was not always a given for Richard. When he was able to do it, he considered it a personal victory over his nerves.

They were both tired from the hike and the extracurricular activity, so they hopped in bed and took a nap. Richard fell asleep right away but woke up 15 minutes later in a cold sweat. He looked at his watch: almost 4:30, only 2½ hours till race time. He checked his pulse rate: 105 beats per minute.

He tried to settle himself down by taking some deep breaths but it didn't help. Lying in Susan's bed, the reality of the situation finally hit him. "Holy shit! I have to actually run this thing."

A wave of nausea came over him and he quickly threw the sheets off him and got out of bed. In doing so he woke Susan.

"What's the matter, babe?" she asked in a sleepy voice. "Gotta go. Gotta get ready," he said. He couldn't even speak in complete sentences anymore, and probably wouldn't be able to until after the ordeal was over.

"Do you want me to come get you and take you to the Dome?" she asked.

"Sure," he said as he was putting on his shoes. He bolted out the front door and heaved a big sigh of relief when he got outside to the fresh air. He hopped in his car and sped away.

He felt tired and wanted to nap longer, but his body would no longer allow that. He had to admit, though, that he was feeling better since he left the apartment. He had a purpose: get ready to kick ass. That sense of purpose settled him down and allowed him to burn off some of that never-ending supply of nervous energy. As long as he could keep himself busy and moving he'd be fine. But if he ran out of things to do before the race, which he knew would eventually happen, his heart would take off like a Concorde jet.

When he got home, he walked in his room, and threw everything he needed into his track bag: spikes, uniform and an extra T-shirt. He put on his racing shorts, his warm-up T-shirt that he wore before every race, his running shoes and his sweat suit—it was starting to get chilly outside.

After he filled up his water bottle he looked at his watch: almost 5 p.m. He called Susan and told her to come over as soon as possible if she wanted to take him. He was ready.

Susan drove up 20 minutes later. During the time he was waiting for her, Richard did exactly what he didn't want to do—he sat in front of the TV and allowed his nerves to tear him up inside. He got up three times to go to the bathroom. But there was hope. Susan was on her way, and he was finally going to lift this dark cloud from over his head. And whether he finished first or last, the dark cloud, he decided, would be gone after the race was over.

When he heard Susan beep her horn, he leaped off the couch. He was eager to leave. He walked down the short hallway to the front door. As he opened the door, he paused and thought: The next time I enter this apartment, I will be a different person. I will know either the great joy of victory, or the crushing disappointment of defeat.

He closed the door and took the next step toward his destiny.

When he got to the Dome it was 5:30 p.m. He parted ways with Susan and checked in with Devlin, to let him know he was alive. He put his stuff down where the team was sitting in the stands. He still had a half-hour until he needed to start warming up, so he sat for a while and watched the meet.

The Dome track was the best in the country. Sprinters loved it because of the wide turns and the hard bouncy surface—great for racing. Distance runners loved it because of the air quality. The air at most indoor track facilities is completely dry and stagnant, which often makes it tough for distance runners to breathe. Richard would usually hack, cough and spit during, and long after, most indoor races. At the Dome though, he didn't have that problem—partly because of the airflow that held up the bubble roof and also because of the mild humidity created by the swimming pool on the level below the track. All of Richard's best indoor times came at the Dome. He hadn't lost a race there in two years.

At five minutes before 6 p.m., Richard started moving toward the stairs. On his way out the door, he passed the results sheets of the races already run. He found the men's 5000 results and saw that Terry Johnson had beaten David Allen again, this time by half a second. Jim Bird was third, and all the way back in sixth was Mad Dog. Mad Dog had actually run his best time of the season, but his place scored only one point for the team. Anthony did even worse, finishing out of the scoring in eighth. Devlin had been hoping for a third place—six points— from Mad Dog and maybe a fifth (worth two points) from Anthony.

The bad news continued as Richard's eyes moved to the sheet that read "Men's Mile: Heat One."

On that sheet he saw the names of his two major competitors: Seamus Rourke and Jon Hines. Both were world class milers who'd be doubling in the 3000. Both had finished in the top ten at the NCAA Cross Country Championships. And both ran for Arkansas.

As he read the results of their mile heat he saw that they both had an easy time. They finished 1-2, running a pathetically slow 4:12.

Richard was mildly disappointed. He had hoped that the other runners would make those two work a little harder and perhaps take away an extra step that would help him. But seeing the times, he realized that they would be practically fresh for the 3000. They would sit on Richard and attempt to outsprint him over the last quarter-mile. The pressure was definitely on Richard to make the race. He had a faster kick than most distance runners in the country. But if he jogged with these boys, he'd get his doors blown off.

Both Rourke and Hines had used their speed to make the last World Championships 1500-meter final—Rourke for Ireland and Hines for Canada. Both had mile times that were eight seconds faster than Richard. A rush of nausea came over him. He knew he had his work cut out for him, especially after the disappointing results in the 5K.

Once he was outside he gave his legs a good shake and he was off on his warm-up. His legs felt heavy on the two-mile jog, but he'd learned that how one feels on a warm-up has absolutely nothing to do with how well one will race.

At the end of the warm-up run he was tired and out of breath. "How am I going to run fast if I feel this shitty right now?" he asked himself.

The tide of doubt was beginning to roll in. His nerves had completely sapped his energy. He would choke for sure and prove to everyone that he was not ready for prime time.

He came back inside the Dome, sat on the carpet and began to stretch. In the middle of a hamstring stretch, Devlin patted him on the shoulder and sat beside him.

"How's it goin', Rickey-boy?" he asked.

Devlin was the last person Richard wanted to see before a big race. Devlin was famous for giving stupid race strategies. Devlin spewed out all the old, worn-out lines, such as, "Just relax, and go out there and compete."

Richard did his best to ignore him, and when asked a question he would only give the standard one-word answer. Finally, Devlin left. Richard was alone—which was the way he wanted it—just as he would be alone in the race. Sure, there were guys from other schools who were good. But Richard knew that when push came to shove, the race would come down to two or three Arkansas Razorbacks and one FIT Aggie.

After he had a good 10-minute stretch, Richard went to the official's table and checked in. When they asked him who he was, he pointed at his name. No words were spoken. He was in mute mode.

Fifteen minutes before the start, they let the competitors in the 3000 onto the track. Richard put on his spikes and did some sprints along the backstretch of the track. He felt better than he did on the warm-up, but he still felt heavy.

He went to the bathroom one more time, and when he came out he got in a few more strides before they called the runners over to the starting line.

Richard stared at the faces of some of the guys in his race. They all had that pasty white, death look with glazed eyes. He knew they were all about as nervous as he was now. But he wondered if any of them were as nervous as he was the previous night. Probably not, he figured. Looking at their faces— faces that had the look of impending doom—made Richard even more nervous. If he was near a toilet or a sink he might have thrown up, but at the starting line he was able to control the nausea.

They were all there: Richard, five Arkansas guys, and about 10 others from various schools. In less than 10 minutes, the race would be run and the agony would be over.

A short time later, John Jenkins, the head official, said, "Runners to your mark." Richard toed the line and looked despairingly at Jenkins, who gave Richard a confident wink. Then the gun fired and the race was under way.

Lifting The Dark Cloud

Richard pushed, shoved and elbowed his way into a position on the right shoulder of the leader—one of the Arkansas no-names. If he let any Arkansas guy control the pace, he was through. The Arkansas runners had the same race plan—jog the first 13 laps, run the 14th and sprint the 15th lap. This way they could save as much energy as possible for the mile final the next day—which all five had qualified for as well.

Richard decided if they were going to beat him, they were going to have to run hard for 15 laps, not for one or two. So 70 meters into the race he made the commitment and took the lead. As he passed the Arkansas leader, Richard heard him say, "Keep dreaming, Dubin."

Richard gave no response to the comment, which neither angered nor intimidated him. And when he took the lead the pace picked up dramatically.

Richard let out a big sigh when he got up front. He felt free and in the clear to run his own race without worrying about tripping on someone else's heels or having his stride cut off. He controlled the race now.

Richard missed his time on the first lap, but he heard his split for the second—61 seconds at 400 meters.

"Holy shit!" he thought. "I feel great and I'm on pace to hit the mile in 4:04."

He relaxed and concentrated on his smooth form and hit the four-lap mark—800 meters—in 2:04. Sixty-three seconds for the second 400 was closer to the pace he expected to run.

His next two 400 splits were both 64, which added up to a 4:12 mile—by far the fastest he'd ever gone out in a 3,000. He felt great, but he wondered if he could hold the other guys off till he crossed the finish line.

Out of curiosity, he looked over his left shoulder as he rounded the first curve after the start/finish line. He could feel that the pack wasn't right on his heels, but he expected to see them only a second or two behind him. Looking back, he saw more daylight back to the second runner than he'd expected. Richard had about a seven-second lead. And judging how they looked compared to how he felt, he was confident that lead would only get larger.

A huge smile broke out on Richard's face. The race was little more than half over, but already the winner had been decided. He took a few seconds to let the victory sink in, and continued to forge ahead. Great days like this didn't come along too often. He wanted to run as fast as he could. An eight-second win would be nice, but not if he could win by 12. He wanted to show those assholes from Arkansas who was boss. And the bigger the win, the wider he could smile at that no-name who told him to "Keep dreaming."

As Richard was enjoying the last seven laps, his senses became heightened. The usual race deafness that kept him from hearing shouts of encouragement was now gone. He could hear the crowd on the upper level chanting something. It was "Dick! Dick! Dick!" And then on the next lap they started chanting "Dubin! Dubin! Dubin!" After that he heard "Aggies! Aggies! Aggies!"

The chants filled Richard with a mid-race adrenaline he had never experienced before. That shot kept him going until he reached $1\frac{1}{2}$ miles (12 laps). But by then it didn't matter, he had only three laps to go, he could just chug it in from there.

He was tired and his pace slowed over the last three laps, but he still ran 7:55.23—a school, Dome and SEC record, as well as the nation's fastest time of the year. He raised his hands as he crossed the finish line and the crowd's roar was deafening.

As soon as he crossed the line, he stopped and turned

around to see how the rest of the race would unfold. He watched in delight as his friend (and occasional steeplechase nemesis), Joe Hall of Auburn, outkicked Rourke and Hines of Arkansas. Hall ran 8:05.78. Richard hugged him when he crossed the finish line, and then went on his victory lap.

As he rounded the inside of the track, he waved to the crowd and looked to see who was up there leading the crazy chants. He found the culprits sitting on the backstretch. It was his friends: Johnny, Hargrove, Phil, Atlas, Gopher, and Jeff. Susan was also sitting with them and cheering loudly. Knowing his friends, this was no surprise to Richard. At closer look, though, he spotted someone who he was very surprised to see. Marie Wyznewski, his old roommate, had come down from Detroit. He looked up at Marie in amazement and pointed to her in a way that said, "I'll see you later."

As Richard's victory lap continued he rounded the second curve and saw where the Razorback team was sitting. He saw the rest of their distance crew sitting in the stands. He stared straight at them and raised his hands to show them who was champion of the distance runners. They may win the meet as a team, but they weren't going to do it by winning any race Richard was running.

He had all the confidence in the world circling the track after the race. Only a few knew what he'd gone through before it.

Richard put his arms down. He looked ahead and saw Devlin sprinting toward him. Richard stopped to prepare for the collision. When they met, Devlin picked Richard up off the ground and bearhugged him. They walked down the homestretch together. Devlin told him, "You did it. You kicked their asses."

Richard knew and responded with a positive nod. All of a sudden, he felt the need to be by himself. They shook hands and Richard headed for the exit door beyond the finish line. He walked to the steps that lead to the third level and sat down to contemplate what had just occurred. Just then he heard a voice call his name.

The dark cloud was gone. And now that the ordeal was over, he knew this would be his only chance to be alone all night. Once his friends caught up with him, he would have no choice but to be with people. Not that he didn't want to spend time with his friends—especially Marie, who came all the way from Michigan—he just wanted that moment alone to reflect on a great achievement, like every champion. So he ignored the voice, hoping it would go away. But it didn't.

The voice called to him again, and he had no choice but to acknowledge it. He looked up and saw that it was John Jenkins, the head official. Seeing Old Man John made Richard forget that he even wanted to spend a moment alone. Spending a moment with Jenkins was even better.

Jenkins sat down next to Richard and said, "I don't want to take up much of your time, Richard. I just wanted to congratulate you in person. I took one look at you at the starting line, and I wasn't sure if you were gonna make it to the finish line. . . let alone win the damn thing and break a bunch of records."

Richard smiled and opened up to Jenkins. "After last night and the day I had today, I wasn't too sure either, Uncle John."

Jenkins put his arm around Richard and said, "I know we officials like to make these meets look real important, but in the larger scope of things they're really not. This ain't life or death you're competing for, son. You're gonna burn out if you don't lighten up a little. Winning ain't no fun when you've spent the previous 24 hours making yourself sick over it."

"I know."

Déjà Vu

Richard found Susan waiting for him as he came out of the interview room. She gave him a big hug, and as they walked out of the Dome toward her VW, she described how good he looked throughout the entire race.

As she talked, Richard was off in a dream land. He wasn't reliving the glory of the moment. He just couldn't stay focused on anything she said.

When they reached her car, he remembered he hadn't done any post-race cool-down. Even though he won the big one, his meet wasn't over. He still had to run the 4x800 relay the next day, and a bad performance in that event would take some of the luster away from his performance in the 3000. He threw his stuff in her car and told her to meet him at his place. He ran off into the night.

It felt good to be alone, running on a cool night. He sighed deeply in the middle of his run when he realized that he would actually get some sleep that night.

Ten minutes later, he walked into his house and saw Susan and Gopher sitting on the couch. Richard asked Gopher what was going on that night, and Gopher mentioned a party at Phil and Atlas's house.

"When does it start?" Richard asked.

"It's started already," Gopher replied.

"Marie's there, isn't she?"

"Yep."

Richard shook his head and contemplated the situation. He wanted to go out to dinner with Susan, but he wanted to see Marie as well. Decisions.

"I have an idea," he said to Susan in his best salesman's pitch. "Let's go over to Phil's, hang out for a bit—maybe a half-hour—and then go to dinner. What do you say?"

"Why don't you go over there and hang out with your friends. I'll wait here and then we'll go out to dinner."

"Phil's your friend, too. Why don't you come with me so we can go straight to dinner from Phil's, instead of having me come all the way back here to pick you up?"

"The place I want to eat is down by the mall. You'll have to pass by Tahiti to go there anyway."

"Why don't you just come with me. Spend some time with me and my friends?" The anger was building inside Richard.

"Because I'm not in the mood to be around a bunch of people tonight," she said.

"Why can't you just say what you're really thinking, Susan," Richard said, raising his voice. "It's not just any bunch of people you don't want to be around tonight. You don't want to be around *my* friends any night because you don't want people to think we're anything more than a platonic relationship. You're afraid you'll be labeled The Girlfriend," he said, holding his fingers up like quotation marks to reinforce the last two words.

"That's right," she said raising her voice in response to his. "I don't want to be labeled anything or belong to anyone. It was that way with Hanson. It was always Hanson and Susan. It could never just be me. I never want that to happen again."

"First of all," Richard fired back, "don't compare anything from your deceased marriage to your relationship with me. We ain't married, and I show you a heck of a lot more respect than your husband ever did. But I gotta be honest, Susan. You talk about, 'It was never just me.' Well, that's the way marriage is, babe. It's the giving up of you as an individual to be a part of something better - a team. All this 'ME, ME, ME' shit is probably the reason your marriage failed."

"Fuck you!" she screamed. "You don't know shit about my marriage and you've got a lot of nerve criticizing it."

"Hey, babe, you're the one that brought it up, not me," he said. "You know, Susan, I just realized this whole conversation is total déjà vu going back to the SEC cross country meet. We do something spectacular. It's time to celebrate a little with friends, and you don't want any part of it. It hurt me in the fall. And it hurts me even more now, because I had hoped that our relationship had moved beyond these little games of yours."

With that comment, Susan picked herself up and ushered herself out the door with the words, "I'm out of here."

As he heard her VW pull away, Richard let out a loud scream of frustration. "FUCK!"

Reasserting Control

Richard didn't sleep nearly as well as he thought he would that night—less than seven hours. He attributed it to the fact that it was an emotional day on all fronts. Between the pre-race desperation and depression and his post-race euphoria, and then his frustration and anger over the argument with Susan, he'd experienced large mood swings that day. And he hadn't had much time to unwind before hitting the sack that night.

Richard was never one to cry over things that were out of his control—and sleep was something that was often out of his control. He awoke at 9 and lay in bed for over an hour before he finally admitted that his body would sleep no more.

He went to the kitchen, but found he wasn't hungry. It was a mystery to him why his hunger hadn't returned after the race. Then like an acid flashback, he remembered the midnight venture he took to the all-you-can-eat breakfast place with Marie and Phil. When he remembered that grease-infested chow session, he understood why he felt hung over despite drinking only one beer.

He took it easy on his body and had a bagel with margarine, which went down a lot easier than it did the day before.

While eating the bagel and watching TV, the phone rang. He answered it with his mouth half-filled with bagel. It was Susan, crying into Bagelville's pay phone.

"What the fuck happened last night?" she said through her tears.

"The same that thing happens every time I suggest a game plan, Susan. You say no. Usually, I acquiesce to your agenda because I don't care what we do. But last night I wanted to do things my way for a change. Is that so wrong?"

"It wasn't wrong until you started in on the personal attacks. What kind of friend says shit like that? You know, I invested a lot of time, energy and emotion in you yesterday. And to end the evening like that was such a downer. Especially after all we went through together yesterday."

Her words hung there for a second or two before he said anything. He'd forgotten in all his selfishness of the day before, that she, too, had been through and seen a lot. She deserved better than the treatment she'd received the night before.

"I'm sorry," he said. He still couldn't contain his anger, though. "But sometimes you make me so fucking mad, it drives me up a wall."

"Well, then maybe we shouldn't see each other any more," she said. It was not the first time she'd made this suggestion.

"Is that what you really want?" he asked, hoping she didn't.

"No. But if you can't handle the relationship the way it is, then maybe we should end it," she said.

She was reasserting control of the relationship, stripping him of the reins he had tried to take last night. He recognized it immediately. But he was powerless to stop her because he was so in love with her.

He bit his lip and agreed to take the relationship in its current state over the unbearable thought of none at all. They agreed to meet at her place that night and they said good-bye.

As he slammed down the receiver, the phone, which was screwed tightly into the wall, came crashing to the floor along with bits of sheetrock.

3

The First Failure

After his impressive performance at the SEC meet, Richard's indoor season ended in disappointment.

On the last day of the SEC meet, Richard's 4x800 relay team won their race. Richard was given the Commissioner's Trophy as meet MVP. But Arkansas walked away with the prize Richard really wanted—the team championship trophy. It was a narrow victory for the Razorbacks, but a victory nonetheless. It was Richard's first experience with failure that year.

The failure did come with some minor rewards, though. The Arkansas runners had newfound respect for Richard after the SEC Indoors. They now knew he was a force to be reckoned with.

It was at the NCAA Indoor Championships in Indianapolis, one week later, where he suffered his first legitimate failure as an individual that year. There, he ran four races: the trials of the 3,000 and 4x800 on Friday, and the finals in both on Saturday. Trials in both events—combined with the tough performance at SECs the week before—proved to be too much for him.

Coming into NCAAs, Richard was considered one of the favorites in the 3000, as he had the fastest time in the country. But when the big boys picked up the pace in the last few laps, Richard withered. Try as he might, he couldn't hang on to the lead pack. His gas tank was empty. He collapsed at the finish line in eighth place. His time was 8:07.42.

He came back in the 4x800, and gutted out a 1:53.7 on the third leg to help the relay squad take fifth. He found it much easier running the 800 tired, as opposed to the 3000.

Arkansas won the meet with 52 points. FIT was second with 42. Richard collected two All-American awards for his efforts. But he knew that his eighth place finish—which scored no points for the team—combined with a mediocre performance on the relay, may have cost his team the championship. After the meet, Devlin made it his business to assign blame in front of the whole team.

"I just want you to know that it wasn't coaching," he said, looking at Richard. "You were ready to go. And you proved it last week. You just pulled a choke job here."

Devlin didn't say outright that he cost the team the championship. But from the speech and the silent treatment Richard received after the speech, he might as well have said it.

Richard stood there looking at the ground as Devlin verbally assaulted him. He said nothing, recalling all the reasons why he couldn't stand Devlin. At first, he felt bad about blowing up in the 3000 and costing his team needed points. But after Devlin's humiliation speech, Richard decided to hold his head high as a way of silently saying, "I did the best I could. So fuck off!"

Richard was reassured by all his teammates after the meet. Some told him he had a great season, and that he alone couldn't have been expected to make up all ten points. He knew, however, that a second-place finish in the 3000 and a third-place finish in the relay would have added 12 points to the team score. Still others cursed Devlin's name. A few said almost exactly what he was thinking, "You did the best you could, Dick. The Devil can go fuck off!"

Richard spent the entire night after the meet drinking alone at the hotel bar. Some of his teammates had tried to get him to go out and have a good time. He wanted none of it. As beer after beer went down his throat that night, his anger toward his coach and himself became more deep-seated. He didn't sleep that night and didn't speak a word to anyone on the flight home. Indianapolis was a miserable experience, and the sooner he got out of that city, the sooner he could forget what had occurred—or so he hoped.

Richard felt better about himself when he got back to Arboretum. His relationship with Devlin, however, was forever changed. On the plane ride home he decided that he could no longer be friends with Devlin. From now on, his relationship was of the coach/athlete variety and nothing more. If he can't take the bad with the good, then he ain't much of a friend or a coach, he told himself. Or a human being, for that matter.

With that situation clearly defined, he could get on to more important things, like running fast in the outdoor season to make up for Indianapolis.

Sending a Message

It was as if Mother Nature herself knew that indoor track season was over. The temperature bolted to a humid 75° only a week later.

While most of the rest of the country was still feeling the fury of March's winter lion, Richard should have been basking in the lamby warmth of Florida. This year was different, though, and Richard was not happy about the change. Mother Nature had turned up the thermostat without warning him.

The usually comfortable late-March weather had departed and was replaced by much warmer weather. Temperatures reached the mid 80's throughout the last two weeks of March and the first week of April, making 3 p.m. workouts much more difficult. Richard was used to dealing with the warmth. After all, this was Florida—land of heat and humidity. He knew that eventually the heat wave would break—or so he hoped—and there would be cooler temperatures for a few weeks before the real heat started in May. He just wanted the temperate March climate to last a little longer than it had.

The weather was only part of the reason Richard was in bad spirits. Devlin had been busting his balls on the track since they returned from Indianapolis. Devlin seemed to be thinking that if he worked Richard to the bone three or four days a week, then he could somehow guarantee that Richard would have a good performance at NCAAs, and therefore prove to the nation that he was a good distance coach.

Although he disagreed with Devlin's method, Richard took his punishment quietly until the Aggie Relays rolled around in the first week of April.

The Aggie Relays Carnival was the state's largest track meet, the nation's fifth largest. Every high school with a track program within 300 miles of Arboretum came to the Relays. There were many who traveled even longer distances than that.

The Relays also attracted some of the best college and open athletes in the country. With the college and open divisions combined, every event had national class athletes, and many had world class athletes. The warm weather didn't hurt in convincing many top athletes to come down for a weekend of sun, fun and a little early season competition.

The week of the Relays, Richard did a track workout on Tuesday. He competed in the 5000 meters Thursday evening and the 1500 meters Saturday afternoon.

In the 5K, Richard shared the lead with Mad Dog for the first two miles. With a mile to go, Mad Dog stepped up the pace, which was slow to begin with, and left Richard. In the last mile, Mad Dog put 10 seconds on Richard—who had little energy before, during or after the race.

Richard said little to Devlin after the race. He didn't want to simply tell Devlin he was exhausted from the heat, the work-outs and the lack of break between indoor and outdoor. He wanted to send a more powerful message. So on Saturday, Richard set out to show him.

When the gun went off Saturday afternoon to start the 1500, Richard pushed and elbowed until he got his favorite spot—just behind the shoulder of the leader. As the pack went by the homestretch grandstand, which was jammed with 5,000 spectators, he heard the announcer say, "Currently running in second is Richard Dubin, an SEC record holder, All-American and one of the greatest distance runners in Florida Tech history."

The crowd applauded loudly, acknowledging Richard's presence. He couldn't help but smile at the performance they were going to witness that day from "one of the greatest distance runners in Florida Tech history."

Richard wasn't sure what the split was for the first 400 meters, but he knew it must have been slow because the pace picked up drastically on the second lap. He tried to stay with the pack, but he couldn't. He felt like he was running with leg weights. He watched helplessly as the pack left him—just as he thought they would.

When he came through the 800 mark he heard his time: 2:05. He shook his head in frustration, but there was nothing he could do. His body could go no faster.

On the last lap, Richard sprinted as hard as he could, mostly to convince himself—and Devlin—that he was trying his hard-est. He knew that "lack of effort" was going to be the first thing Devlin would look at when evaluating his performance. Therefore, he had to put on a good show.

Going down the homestretch, Richard, who was one place ahead of the caboose, received what is every distance runner's worst nightmare—the sympathy clap.

The sympathy clap happens at the end of the race when the last place runners are finishing up. It's the crowd's way of saying, "You stink, but we appreciate your effort today. So here's a little parting gift for you."

Richard would always argue with sprinters that distance running is a tougher sport than the sprints because of the "embarrassment factor." The sympathy clap was a large part of that.

Even with his half-hearted effort at the end, Richard crossed the line in 3:58, which equates to a 4:15 mile—his slowest performance since his alcoholic days.

Devlin pulled Richard aside almost immediately after he finished. "What the fuck was that?" Devlin said, choosing the direct route rather than beating around the bush.

"That was all I had today," said Richard, who'd rehearsed his response. Devlin, however, was not convinced.

"That's bullshit, Rickey. The way you've been kickin' ass in workouts, you're gonna tell me that was all you had?"

Richard restrained himself from flying off the handle. A loud tone of voice never went over well with Devlin. So he said in a soft, yet forceful voice, "I haven't been kicking ass in workouts. I've been struggling every day since SEC Indoors. Shit, Devlin, I ran six races in two weeks. I was exhausted after indoor season. But you gave me no break. I've been on the track six out the past 12 days. I got nothing left. Can't you see that? You think I want the sympathy clap? When I embarrass you as a coach, I also embarrass me as an athlete. You think I want that?"

"You sayin' this whole thing is my fault?" Devlin said with a ton of defensiveness.

"I'm not assigning blame, Devlin," he said calmly. He had to continue to remind himself not to go ballistic. "I'm just saying I need a rest. Now you can either continue to work me into the ground and get mediocre results, like my two races this weekend, or you give me some time to recover. What do you say?"

"I say this isn't the time or the place to discuss this matter," said Devlin, now trying to play the mature, level-headed coach. "Come to my office on Monday and we'll talk about it. In the meantime, get yourself an easy run tomorrow."

Richard smiled as he left the track. The plan had worked. The message had been received.

The Nude Relay

Competition was definitely one factor that attracted athletes to the Aggie Relays. Another factor that made athletes, particularly men, want to compete in the Aggie Relays was the party afterwards. Of particular interest was the race held Sunday at 2 a.m. after the relay party. The race was known widely as the Nude Relay.

The Nude Relay, now in its fifth year, had taken on an identity all its own—as with anything that takes on cult status. Whether there was an official party or not, word of mouth over the years had guaranteed that people were going to show up at the FIT track at 2 a.m. on the last night of the Aggie Relays.

The Nude Relay, and the party that preceded it, had become so popular, that anyone caught wearing "FIT Track" paraphernalia at the Aggie Relays would be bombarded with questions about where and when the party would be.

Richard attempted to fix that problem by not wearing anything that said FIT, except when he raced. But anyone that knew anything about the Nude Relay knew that Richard was the man in charge. So it almost didn't matter what he wore. If Richard wanted to concentrate on his upcoming race, he couldn't be anywhere near the track stadium on the last day of Aggie Relays.

University officials considered the event, and the hubbub surrounding it, to be an embarrassment. There had been numerous attempts in years past to halt the event—by the president of the university, the campus police, and Devlin himself. All were unsuccessful.

Every year, Devlin would give a speech before Aggie Relays week about partying and staying out of trouble with the law. "In particular, a certain party that occurs every year around this time," he would say, never referring to it by name.

He would threaten to kick people off the team if they were caught with their pants down, suspend others if they were caught drinking at the party, and issued other idle threats that would scare the freshmen for a few days until they wised up.

In the end, Devlin knew there was nothing he could do, unless he intended to suspend every sprinter, thrower, and distance runner on the team, from the studs on down to the walk-ons. For one night a year, the entire FIT track team—as well as most of the athletic program—could be found at one place: the Nude Relay Bash.

The Nude Relay was created during Richard's freshman year at the Aggie Relays party—a blowout held at Johnny and Hargrove's Crackhouse. As the party wound down, the two inebriated hosts had a crazy idea—normal, actually, considering the source.

"Let's go down to the track and run a nude quarter," they said. Those who were left at the party—Richard, Jeff, Phil and some of his biker friends, along with Atlas and some of the swimmers, loved the idea. A tradition was born.

This year, Richard and his roommates were hosting it. Richard and Marie had hosted it the past three years when they lived at Tahiti #312.

Richard loved hosting a party when he lived with Marie because he knew that, between the two of them, things would run smoothly. Beer and loud music would be requisitioned, the party would be properly policed, and they would both be up the next day cleaning the place and returning to LBP—Life Before Party—as quickly as possible.

He was not nearly as confident in his current roommates, especially when it came to cleaning up. He had a feeling going in that it was mostly up to him to pull this shindig off. But he had the experience in these affairs to pull it off, and to their credit and his surprise, his roommates followed through with the responsibilities he delegated to them.

One problem that seemed to grow bigger—or smaller—every year, was the collection of funds. Richard considered The Nude Relay Bash to be a party put on by the FIT distance runners, not just the people hosting the party. So Richard would go around asking the other distance runners for five- or ten-dollar donations. Few gave until the night of the party, and even then they gave less than they were supposed to.

Richard hated asking other people for contributions. One reason was that he felt like he was asking for a handout, which made him uncomfortable. Another reason was that he was one of only two Jews on the team—Jeff being the other. He didn't like the image of having the Jew manage the money. It was too stereotypical.

Every year Richard would ask someone else to handle the collection of funds. But either that person would say no, or they simply would neglect to do it.

"Face it Dick. You're the best when it comes to this stuff. You're the only one that can do it," Gopher would say as he gave his reasons for refusing the job.

It was true that Richard was the best at organizing the parties and collecting funds. But that image of the team Jew coming around asking for money left a bad taste in his mouth, even though the money was going to a good cause. In all his time down in Arboretum, Richard was never able to remove the religion chip from his shoulder.

Another problem that had the organizers hamstrung in their preparation for the party was their phone. When Richard returned home from his abysmal performance in the 1500, he wanted to call Phil and Atlas. He wanted to use their empty beer kegs and taps rather than put the $100 for the deposit on his credit card. Unfortunately, the phone was not working.

Not sure if it was the telephone or the phone company, he went to the next door neighbor's apartment to call Southern Bell. Ma Bell told him the bill hadn't been paid in over two months. Even if it was paid immediately, the phone couldn't be reconnected until Monday.

Richard was responsible for collecting money for every bill in the house—rent, electricity, and cable—except the phone. That was Gopher's responsibility because it had been put in his name when he moved into The Clubhouse two years before.

Gopher was late in paying the phone bill every month. In December, his procrastination incurred a $26 late fee. Gopher actually had the nerve to complain about paying the late fee himself. This current disconnection came at a particularly bad time, though.

Richard wanted to strangle Gopher when he realized what had happened. Yet he needed Gopher to get the party off the ground. So when he saw Gopher and Jeff, he simply informed them of the telephone screw-up matter-of-factly.

"Hey, I need you guys to go pick up the empty kegs from Phil and Atlas's. Oh, and by the way, the phone's been disconnected because Gopher didn't pay the bill."

Richard was hoping this latest revelation would cause Jeff to get angry and join him in condemning their irresponsible roommate. It didn't work. The two laughed so hard, Richard wasn't sure if they were laughing at Gopher or at him. Eventually, Richard couldn't help but crack a smile. But he was still pissed off.

Despite Richard's concerns, the group moved efficiently and the party was ready to go at 6 p.m.

Richard and Jeff sat on the puke couch. They drank from the first of the kegs to be tapped, and watched the NCAA basketball tournament on TV. After a long and hectic day, it was their one chance to relax for an hour before the madness started.

They exchanged pleasantries in mocking imitation of their fathers—who drank coffee, smoked cigarettes and discussed their sons every Sunday morning at Gary's Coffee Shop in Fresh Meadows, New York. Usually Jeff's father would talk about what Richard was doing, and Richard's father would offer up tidbits about Jeff. This is the way they got their information about their children.

"So, is Susan coming tonight?" Jeff asked, taking a drag from his imaginary cigarette.

"What do you think?" Richard snapped.

"What's up with that shit?"

"It's her way of keeping the relationship on her terms. 'Not tonight' has become her battle cry."

"Don't worry about it," Jeff said. "We'll have fun tonight."

"Hey, you won't catch me with my head down. Unless, of course, I'm passed out," Richard said.

By 8 p.m. most of the hard-core groupies of the Nude Relay were there. Phil and Atlas along with about half the swim team and a few bikers were performing nude handstands on the keg, timing how long each person could hold the flowing tap to his mouth before having to come down. Jeff and Richard sat back and watched the madness that would only increase as the evening grew older.

A few minutes later, Hargrove walked in the door wearing three items: black Converse All-Star high tops, a black cape, and a black sock over his penis. When he came inside he didn't stop to be admired. He walked straight back to the porch. Without saying a word, he elbowed aside the swimmer who was next in line for a kegstand, went upside down and swallowed for 58 seconds. He received high-fives from Phil and Atlas, both of whom were now completely in the buff.

Hargrove shook his head to get the cobwebs out and went over to talk to Jeff and Richard, who were watching from the puke couch in awe. A closer look revealed he had something

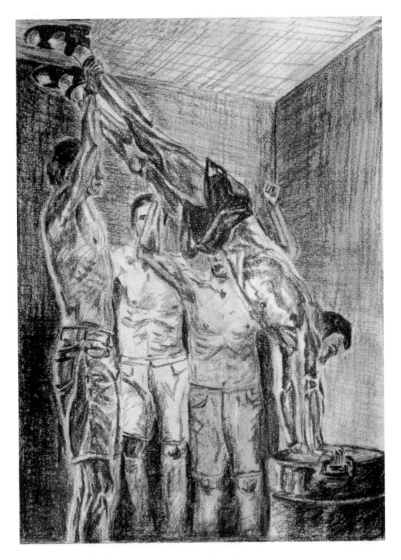

written on his chest:

"GIVE ME NUDITY OR GIVE ME HEAD!"

"How's it going, fellas?" Hargrove said, standing with his feet shoulder-width apart and his arms crossed. With the cape, he looked like a sexually demented superhero.

Richard envisioned a misguided hero who flew around the world in search of evil-doers. With his super-powerful penis, which could grow to six feet long and shoot lasers, all he had to do was point his hips in the direction of evil and his cock would do the rest. Of course, allowing your smaller head to do all the thinking had its disadvantages. Sometimes, while in pursuit of evil, a beautiful woman would cross his path and the high-speed chase would take on a whole new meaning. But he meant well, and he was very popular with the ladies. No, it wasn't Steven J. Hargrove, Jr. It was the MAD COCK SOCKER!

"I see you're getting down to business right away," Richard said. "No hesitation there."

"That's correct, Boy Blunder," he said in a superheroic voice.

"Where's Johnny?" Richard asked.

"He's doing his pre-Relay mental preparation. He takes this event pretty seriously, you know. He hasn't lost in five years. I'm kind of worried about him, though. He said he's had trouble sleeping and eating," said Hargrove, mocking Richard's pre-race problems.

"As long as he doesn't have trouble drinking," Richard said. "You know the rules: Six-beer minimum if you want to be eligible for the relay."

"Don't you worry about my partner in crime," said the Mad Cock Socker. "He was downing six packs long before the best part of you stained the back seat of your grandparents' station wagon. . . and he was doing it the nude too."

"Let me ask you something," Jeff said with feigned seriousness. "If the temperature drops, how's your cock-sock going to stay on?"

"Oh, silly boy," he said. "Not only is the cock-sock bulletproof, it's got a special heating device inside. The rest of my body could be suffering from frostbite and my dick will still be warm enough to get a stiffy." He then broke into a loud villainous laugh, wheeled and broke off for another kegstand, leaving Richard and Jeff in hysterics.

Mad Dog and Gin showed up little while later. Gin was wearing a black long-sleeve shirt, black tights and running shoes that were dyed black. Mad Dog continued the black theme with black jeans, ratty running shoes and a black T-shirt. The T-shirt had a stick figure with its head attached upside down. The words above read: "FIX MY HEAD!"

"You got it?" Richard yelled to Mad Dog as he headed out toward the keg. Mad Dog answered his question by digging out a piece of paper from his front pocket and holding it out for Richard to see. "Good," Richard responded. Mad Dog's special verse would be delivered later on in the evening.

"Sitting on this couch, I feel like a talk show host," Richard said to Jeff. And then he said in his fake announcer's voice, "People Who Are Addicted To Getting Naked. On the next Dick and Jeff show."

"It's rare we get to see such quality as we're seeing tonight," Jeff said.

"Or as we're going to see later," Richard added.

"I predict that wherever we go after college, we will never know people as crazy as the ones we associate with down here," Jeff said.

"Jeff, my friend, I do believe you've hit the nail square on the head," Richard said. "I think the only place I could meet people more insane than our friends down here, would be in a mental institution which, for me, is not entirely out of the question."

By 10:30 p.m. the place was packed wall-to-wall with people. Another few hundred or so were outside. It was by far the largest party Richard had ever hosted. He enjoyed the mob scene, but he definitely preferred the situation four hours earlier: 20 hard-core people drinking and having a good time, without having to shout or wait to use the bathroom. Richard realized, though, that part of having something great like the Nude Relay, was dealing with the masses. He just hoped that most of them would go away before 2 a.m. The Relay was difficult enough to pull off. With nearly 400 people, it was impossible.

Fortunately, the organizing committee—which consisted of Richard, Hargrove, Johnny, Phil, Atlas, Jeff, Gopher and Mad Dog—had a backup plan. They knew the party would be huge, and there would be many hangers-on who would want to be a part of the madness—or just witness it. The committee had been flirting with the idea of ending the Relay tradition as it had evolved, and starting over. They could do this by holding the Relay at a different venue—possibly the golf course. They made the decision to wait to announce where the Relay would be until right before it was time to leave. If there were too many people around, they would tell the riffraff to go to the track. Those in the know would slide across the street to the golf course and run the Relay on a measured 400-meter loop on the cross country course.

Richard found all the media attention the Relay attracted over the last two years to be amusing. Getting notices in every major newspaper in the U.S., as well as the *London Times* and *Sports Illustrated,* was fun at first. But with all of that attention came a lot of trouble that Richard didn't want to deal with; not the least of which was the possibility of having a picture of his bare ass thrown on Devlin's desk Monday morning. He needed to stay out of trouble this year. And if it meant having the media trash the event—which would happen if the founding fathers weren't there to organize it—then so be it. The event was better before the media got hold of it anyway. Destroying the Nude Relay for its own sake seemed a noble aim to the organizing committee.

Richard spent much of the rest of the evening doing what he did best—collecting money for more kegs and going out and getting them. While he didn't like asking for the contributions, he actually liked going and getting the kegs. It helped keep him from getting completely wasted (although he still had plenty to drink and shouldn't have been driving). And when he showed up with the goods, he felt like a saint delivering bread to the starving natives. He was a hero for about 30 seconds.

By 2 a.m. the party had been through eight kegs and was busily draining the ninth. The police had been by the apartment three times telling whomever claimed to live there to keep the noise down and keep the people inside.

The end of the party and the beginning of the march to the Relay site was signified by the reading of Mad Dog's poem. Mad Dog had wanted to read the poem at 1 a.m., but was convinced to wait in hopes that most of the crowd would leave within the next hour or so.

The organizers had hoped that the party would be more subdued by 2 a.m.; maybe 40 or 50 people instead of the 150 that were still standing. It was clear that the backup plan needed to go into effect.

Everyone was herded inside to hear the poem. Mad Dog hopped on a chair and waited for silence. As always, the originals—Richard, Jeff, Gopher, Phil, Atlas and Johnny (who showed up shitfaced at 11 p.m.)—got naked and knelt before Mad Dog. Hargrove, who was holding up surprisingly well considering the amount he'd consumed, stood behind them in superhero pose.

The crowd became silent and Mad Dog said, "This poem is called 'The Nude Relay Goes Straight to Hell.'"

Richard could tell immediately that Mad Dog had taken to heart the idea of the euthanasia of the Nude Relay.

"From the conquest of truth, long battles on end,
A past lost to innocence, no one can amend.
I stand here before you, for one final time,
To bring forth the end, the last naked rhyme.
Now the time is upon us, that one final stage,
To unleash the savage demons, from their eternal cage.
We've laid back on fire and welcomed the pain,
And staggered through fate and its cold bitter rain.
Now disaster is here, it knows its own name;
The day our true victim, the night our forever game.
Now see fires of destruction, scattered through the land,
A savage dragon brings terror, held tight in its hand.
Now with one final charge, the game here must end,
For we've broken all the rules, there's none left to bend.
Now our final naked task, such a long history to tell.
It's time to send the Nude Relay right straight to hell."

The crowd cheered and snickered throughout the poem. . . and let out a roar at the end. "Right straight to hell!"

With 150 people packed into the living room and kitchen, it was impossible to quiet everyone down after the poem was over.

Mad Dog shouted as loud as he could, "I have an announcement. We're going to the track. Let the nude madness begin!"

With that, everyone ran out the door and charged toward any form of transportation that could get them to the track. Richard, Jeff and Atlas started running toward the track, but veered right onto the golf course at the last minute.

They were the first ones to make it to the starting line, which was on the backside of the cross country course on the flat part of the horseshoe loop. They slapped hands and high-fived when they got there.

They began taking off their clothes when the others started showing up. Hargrove, Johnny and Phil came the back way through some thick bushes. A small group of swimmers and runners, including some women, showed up. When all were assembled, Richard counted heads. . . er, bodies. They had a total of 28 runners—a perfect number.

From out of the darkness they heard a shout. "All right,

you're all under arrest!"

They panicked. Most grabbed their clothes and started to dash off. Richard recognized the voice and chuckled. The voice belonged to John Jenkins, the official. Jenkins had started every race at the Aggie Relays for the past 20 years—including the Nude Relay. He wasn't going to miss this one.

When Richard realized that the Relay would not be run at the track, he had called Jenkins to let him know where the race would take place. Being the starter for all FIT cross country meets as well, Jenkins knew exactly where to meet the nudists.

All the distance runners knew the quarter-mile loop; they often ran windsprints on the loop because it was the one flat part of the whole course. Richard explained it to the others. "You run down the fairway to the cone by the last tree and you cut towards the flag on the green. Then you cut to the cone on the other side of the fairway and then dash back home to here," he said pointing at the cone he was standing next to in the middle of the fairway. The diamond-shaped course was easy to see because of the full moon that lit the course.

There were seven teams. Jeff, Gopher, Hargrove and Johnny made up one team. Phil, Atlas, Mad Dog and Richard were another team. The swimmers made up two teams. The distance runners along with a few sprinters made up two other teams. There was also a women's team made up of two swimmers and two distance runners. Gin ran on the team with the male sprinters, who, with her as their anchor leg, were suddenly a serious threat to take the title. It was a well-rounded field, for sure.

Jenkins came prepared, passing out batons to the lead off leg of each team. "All right, let's have big dicks in the front, pencil dicks in the back," he joked, and then held up his starter's pistol. "Now, seriously. . . Runners to your mark. . . Set. . . BANG!"

The team with the two sprinters got out to an early lead, mostly because they weren't as drunk as everybody else. Richard wondered whether they'd even met the six-beer minimum.

Jeff and Phil led off for their respective teams. Phil sat behind Jeff the whole way, never letting him get more than a second or two ahead. The fact that Phil could keep up with Jeff was pretty shocking to Richard. But then he recalled that Jeff didn't hold his beer as well as Phil, and that Jeff had gained 10 pounds and hadn't run a step since he retired from the sport after the cross country season.

Jeff handed off to Gopher, who also hadn't run a step since he quit the team. Richard glanced at his watch—the one article of clothing he'd kept on—and clocked Jeff at a respectable 65 seconds. Less than two seconds later, Phil handed to Atlas, who actually had been running in preparation for the Nude Relay. Atlas, who had shed over five pounds from his nude training, had a good stride and made up the lead on a struggling Gopher.

Richard laughed when he saw what his teammate was doing to Gopher's lead. Gopher would catch a lot of shit for blowing a lead to a retired, overweight swimmer. They came in together. Gopher handed off to Hargrove; Atlas, who ran about 66 seconds for his leg, handed off to Mad Dog.

Hargrove and Mad Dog were the unknown factors in this race. They might run nearly 60 seconds for the quarter-mile (as Hargrove had done two years ago). Or they might run over 90 seconds, as Mad Dog had done last year. It all depended on how much they drank, which even they couldn't keep track of.

Mad Dog went out hard, but Hargrove—going without the cape—hung on tenaciously. They started kicking with about 50 meters to go. Richard couldn't help but laugh at these two naked and wasted distance runners as they sprinted in together and handed off to the anchor legs, one of whom was Richard.

Johnny took the lead and Richard started laughing again when he saw Johnny's jiggling butt. But Richard shook his head and started taking the race seriously when Johnny opened up a scary 15-yard lead. Richard dug down and closed it up. He didn't want to be responsible for his team losing, especially since he'd drunk only seven or eight beers throughout the entire evening. Johnny probably had downed that many before he showed up at the party. Johnny was a tough competitor, though, and had been known to run under 60 when he was so bombed he could barely stand.

Johnny and Richard were moving fast. As they rounded the last cone and turned for the final 120-meter straightaway to the start/finish line, they'd passed several others (including Gin) and were now in the lead. Richard pulled up beside Johnny and prepared himself for the mad dash to the finish.

It didn't matter that they were naked, smashed, and on a golf course at 2:30 a.m. It was two guys duking it out for pride in an event they would have bragging rights to for the next 365 days. This was athletic competition stripped to its core elements.

Richard monitored Johnny's every move in the final stretch. Johnny was quicker than Richard, who feared getting left behind by a surprise move. With 70 meters left, he saw Johnny put his head down and start sprinting. Richard went into a full sprint himself and made up the few steps he lost on Johnny's first move.

Down the fairway, Johnny and Richard battled, the full moon giving the small crowd just enough light to see the action. Fortunately the loop was toward the back nine of the course where no one could hear the crowd screaming as the two approached the finish line with legs, elbows and heads rocking and rolling.

Like all experienced athletes, they both knew exactly where the finish line was, despite the fact that they both had their eyes closed the last 30 meters. They leaned at the finish line and fell down a few steps later. Then the barfing began, an upchuckfest in which almost every other finisher joined soon after.

No one knew for sure who won. Jeff, Gopher, and Hargrove claimed Johnny got the nod. Phil, Atlas, and Mad Dog naturally sided with Richard. John Jenkins, the head official, declared it a tie.

There was a lot of disagreement about who'd won that night. But two things that everyone agreed on were: they'd been treated to a great race, and Richard and Johnny's time of 51.7 (according to Jenkins's watch) had to be some sort of world record for the bare-assed and blotto.

Tornado

After they recovered, the two victorious anchor legs walked on rubbery legs with their teammates back to the apartment. The idea was to celebrate the tie by finishing off the last of the kegs. When they arrived back at The Clubhouse, the door was wide open. They walked in to find the living room destroyed.

The damage to the apartment was extensive. Empty kegs were thrown through the sheetrock walls to expose the brick that separated the apartments. Broken glass from beer bottles covered the carpet. Items such as ketchup, eggs and mayonnaise were removed from the refrigerator and thrown at the walls. Garbage from the kitchen was scattered throughout the apartment.

Richard went in his room to find a few more holes in the wall. He thought it looked like a drunken tornado had struck. The storm had thrown around some empty kegs and took just about everything from the refrigerator, while leaving the TV, VCR and stereo alone.

The upstairs had been spared. Richard figured that whoever was having fun at their expense was probably getting nervous and dashed off before hitting the second floor.

After assessing the damage, Richard started to laugh. "What else can go wrong in this hellhole?" he said out loud.

Phil called 911 from the apartment next door to report the incident. Three hours later—about 6 a.m.—a police car showed up. Out of the car stepped the police officer who had come to the apartment three times that night to tell them to keep the noise down.

The officer had a judgmental look about him as he scanned the walls, which, if they weren't caved in, showed the creative finger-painting done at Dick Stomp six months earlier.

Before making any inquiries, the officer spoke: "I want you to know that I saw what was going on at the party last night, and that I'm going to include it in my report."

They all knew where he was leading. In an effort to save paperwork, he was going to place the blame on the "residents," saying it all occurred during the party.

The group argued with him, saying the party had ended and that they weren't responsible for the damage which took place while they were gone. They neglected to tell him the truth, though, about their exact whereabouts when the incident occurred, however.

At one point, the discussion became so heated that Atlas had to drag Phil outside to keep him from attacking the cop. Phil could be heard outside screaming, "You jelly-donut-eating motherfucker!"

The cop left with his version of the story, while Richard, Jeff and Gopher were left holding the bag. One careless act—forgetting to lock their door—had turned a historic night of frolicking and fun into a nightmare.

Richard stood for a while and just stared at the mess. Looking at the walls, he came to the realization that Tahiti #160 was now unlivable—for him, anyway. It was getting toward the end of the semester, the most important part of the most important track season of his career. This was the season when he was going to shock the world at the NCAAs and Olympic Trials. Yet here he was—this champion distance runner—looking at the caved-in, painted-on walls of his home. It reminded him of a poster his mother had put on the refrigerator when he was a kid. It said, "How can I soar with the eagles, when I'm surrounded by turkeys."

But if Richard was surrounded by turkeys, he knew he had the potential to be one as well. He hung his head and admitted to himself that he'd been one that night for sure. And now he would pay for his stupidity.

In his grand scheme, he'd planned on doing only important things in April: graduating, figuring out what he was going to do with his life, and getting ready for the big meets that were only six weeks away. Now he would have to spend much of his energy moving, finding another place to live and getting out of the lease with Tahiti.

He loathed the act of moving, yet he could never seem to stay in one place for more than a year. He'd moved six times since he'd left home five years earlier, and each time he packed up his belongings he hated the process even more. But it was all part of the college experience; and when he moved to a different place at the start of each year, he counted on at least being settled into his living space nine months later when the heart of the outdoor track season came around.

That wouldn't be the case this year, though. And the more he thought about having to move, the more he became depressed about having to go through the process once more.

But his mind was made up. Staying would only make him more depressed. He knew his limits. He knew he had to get out. He could no longer live in shit. The tough part would be convincing Jeff and Gopher that the damage—despite looking awful—was not so expensive as to make the Tahiti management sue them.

Richard left The Clubhouse and began the preliminary business of moving out—mostly packing up clothing into boxes. He tried to hold his head high, but that image of turkeys—particularly the self-image—would not go away.

He went over to Phil and Atlas's house and called Susan. She opened the door for him at 8 a.m. He was asleep five minutes later.

He dreamed he had a large lead in the final lap of the Olympic Trials steeplechase. But the other competitors were catching up to him because he was slowing down. When he looked down to see why his legs were failing him at such a crucial moment, he noticed there were ropes tied to each leg. On the end of each rope was a turkey. He tried to kick the ropes off his legs without coming to a complete stop. But the more he tried to remove them, the closer his competitors came to passing him. He awoke just as everyone in the race went by him.

When he was fully awake, around noon, he told Susan about the dream. She told him he was shouting "Get away!" in his sleep. He gave her a report on the entire night, and when he told her of his intention to have everything out of The Clubhouse by Sunday, she applauded the idea.

"For your own sanity, you need to get out," she said.

The only question was where was he going to move. If worse came to worse, he could always move back in the athletic dorm, a place he hadn't lived in since his freshman year. He really didn't want to live in the dark, depressing dorm underneath the football stadium. But if that's what it took to get away from Nightmare Central, he'd gladly do it.

He haltingly asked Susan if he could live with her for a little while. She seemed cold to the idea, and even Richard knew that the potential for disaster was great. At that point, he knew only one thing—he'd sleep on any bed, couch, or floor before he'd spend another night at Tahiti #160.

She agreed to let him keep "some things" at her place for a while until he found a permanent place. He went back to Tahiti to begin moving.

On his way back, he stopped over at Phil and Atlas' house to find out how they were feeling after the long, hard night. Phil was the only one at home. Atlas was at his girlfriend Mary's house, where he'd been practically living since January.

Phil intimated to Richard that Atlas planned to move to Tallahassee with Mary after graduation, just three weeks away at the end of April. This left Phil in need of a roommate till the end of the lease, which ended in mid-August. Phil was not happy about his best friend leaving him high and dry, and doing little to help him find a replacement just three weeks before he was planning to ditch.

A huge smile broke out on Richard's face as he told Phil of his plan to leave The Clubhouse immediately. Phil was worried, though, about causing a bad situation between Richard, Gopher and Jeff.

"First of all," Richard said, stating his case, "Jeff is graduating in three weeks. He can stay with someone till the end of the semester and he has almost nothing to store anyway. As for Gopher, I can't see him wanting to live there after what happened this weekend. And it's not as if we have much choice. The management's probably going to evict us after they see the damage. We don't even have a phone any more because that asshole forgot to pay the bill. I can live without a lot of things, Phil. But I can't live in shit and without a phone. I'm not going to be a dick about it. Gopher and Jeff are my friends. I'm going to pay my fair share to get us out of this mess."

"As long as I'm not caught in the middle, I'm down with it," Phil said cautiously.

They shook hands on the deal and agreed to present this idea to Atlas: move to Mary's as soon as possible, or find another roommate. In the meantime, Richard would stay in the athletic dorm until Atlas' room was vacant.

Moving Out

Driving back to Tahiti, Richard was elated and relieved that he'd worked out a living arrangement so quickly. It lifted his spirit out of its depression, but only temporarily.

When he got back to The Clubhouse, he was shocked to see Gopher actually cleaning up the place.

The man hasn't done a bit of house cleaning the entire year, Richard thought. But now that the place is a disaster, he's got a vacuum in his hand.

It seemed such a lost cause at this point; Richard was hoping Gopher had given up, as he did with just about everything else in his life.

"I spoke to the landlady," Gopher said. "She said she wants this month's rent, our security deposit and an extra $600 to fix the holes. Then we can stay."

It was clear that Gopher wanted the exact opposite of what Richard wanted. He wanted to stay through the end of the lease. Richard felt deflated when he realized this. But he was determined to make Gopher see the light.

"Look Gopher. I don't think it's a good idea if we stay here anymore. The landlady can have our $500 security deposit and she's already got our last month's rent that we gave her in August. This way she'll have a whole month to fix up the place enough to rent it to somebody else, and she won't be losing a dime. As for the rest of it, she's just trying to rip us off," Richard said calmly, trying to convince Gopher that leaving made the most sense. "You have three weeks till the end of the semester. Then you were going to go home and work, anyway. Why pay all that money just so you have a place to keep your stuff over the summer?"

"You're just trying to ditch because you're not on the lease," Gopher said in an angry tone. Richard was afraid he would bring up that subject. Officially, Jeff, Gopher and Mad Dog were on the lease. Richard never signed the lease—which was no accident.

When he moved into #160, the four tenants—Gopher, Jeff, Mad Dog and himself—were one more than was legally allowed for Tahiti's three-bedroom townhouses. Therefore, they needed one person to stay off the lease. Since he was the newcomer to the apartment and the apartment was not in the greatest condition when he got there, Richard "agreed" to stay off the lease. It was an agreement he didn't mind at all because it kept him legally separated from the damage that was already there, not to mention the damage that would inevitably come during the year.

When Gopher called him out on that fact, Richard felt ashamed. He understood where his roommate was coming from and tried to allay his fears.

"First of all, we're all friends here," he said, realizing he probably sounded like a used car salesman. But he went on anyway. "I've only known you a couple of years, Gopher. So I could see how you would think that maybe I might ditch and run if I were an asshole—which I'm not. But I've known Jeff all my life. He's like a brother to me. Why would I want to toss away a lifetime friendship over a few hundred dollars? It just doesn't make sense. Just as it doesn't make sense to stay here any longer."

"That's a lovely speech, Dick. But the fact remains that if we leave, they're not going to come after you or Jeff, because you guys are going to be graduated and gone from this place. They're going to come after people they can easily find—like me. Or even worse, my parents. They have their address, you know."

"Gopher, they have enough money between our last month's rent and our security deposit to fix the walls. Maybe they're losing a couple of hundred dollars in lost rent, but they'll get that back from renter's insurance. It will cost them more than five times that amount to hire an agency to find us, and a lawyer to sue us. And if they do sue us—which they won't— they're going to realize we've got no money because we're college students. The management knows this. They're just trying to bully us for as much money as they can get. And it appears to be working on one of us."

"And like I said," Gopher countered, "it's easy to be so sure when your name isn't on the lease."

The two went back and forth—each time getting louder— until Richard said, "Well, if you'd paid the phone bill and did your dishes more than once a semester, I might actually be willing to stay!"

Gopher dropped the vacuum cleaner and the two charged each other. Richard wrestled Gopher to floor. The two put themselves in a dual headlock and were taking turns punching each other on the top of the head with shots that hurt the knuckles much more than the head they connected with.

Jeff, who was coming back from the laundry room, dropped his basket of underwear and mercifully broke up the brawl before someone broke a hand. Without another word, Richard went to his room and began packing. All of his belongings were gone from Tahiti #160 within an hour.

His relationship with Gopher was a lost cause. But he didn't want to lose his friendship with Jeff over his sudden departure. After he finished moving into the athletic dorm, Richard went over to Tahiti to settle things with Jeff. He wanted to call Jeff, but Jeff no longer had a connected phone. And Richard knew it was more effective to settle things face to face.

As usual, Jeff took the middle ground between Gopher and Richard, as he had all year. Richard explained that it didn't make financial sense to stay, and that it was in everyone's best interest to just break the lease.

Jeff saw Richard's point and admitted that it would work best for him as well, being that he would be leaving town a few days after graduation to search for a job in New York. But he also recognized Gopher's fear of being chased by the Tahiti management because he would be the only one among them still in school, which made his address and phone number very easy to find. Jeff also took Richard to task—in his own diplomatic manner—for moving so abruptly and leaving Gopher and Jeff to handle the dirty work by themselves.

Richard defended himself mildly and weakly. He claimed that he couldn't deal with management because he wasn't on the lease—which even he knew was mostly nonsense. Richard also reasoned that they all needed to move as quickly as possible. "The longer we stay," he told Jeff, "the more charges they'll try to stick us with."

In the end though, Richard apologized for the rogue manner in which he handled the situation. He vowed to stick with his former roommates and pay his equal share of whatever they agreed to pay. He also promised to help both of them move and find places to stay until the end of the semester.

Richard left Tahiti Sunday night feeling much better about the situation after the talk with Jeff. He didn't get to resolve things with Gopher. But time would heal those wounds; especially with Gopher, who couldn't hold a grudge more than a day or two.

Richard moved into the athletic dorm that weekend and took over Atlas' room a week later.

2

The Last Straw

Another warm Friday night in North Florida's early May. Richard called Susan at 6 and they made plans to ride bikes to the Downtown Jazz Festival and catch some music in the open air. She told him that he needed to be ready to leave by 8 because one of her favorite local bands would be performing at 8:30.

"I really want to see this band, Richard," she told him over the phone. "So if you don't think you'll be ready when I get over to your place, I'll just meet you downtown."

"Don't worry about me. I'll be ready," he said.

Richard showered, ate and prepared himself for the evening. He sat down on the front porch with a beer in his hand and watched the sun set. He was relaxed and felt mellow. After the sun was down he went inside, sat down on the couch, watched television, and waited for Susan's arrival.

8 p.m. came and went and there was no sign of Susan. You always have to give her a half-hour leeway, he thought. That's just the peril of dating Susan Connor.

8:30 p.m. came and still no Susan. Richard began to stew in anger on the couch. He was really looking forward to attending the Jazz Festival, and not just because he would be with Susan. Richard liked jazz and had even played trumpet in his high school's jazz ensemble.

He thought about leaving her and just going himself, but he was curious as to when she would show. There had been nights that she turned up over an hour late. She always showed, though.

Phil, now his new roommate, put it best: "When you're dealing with Susan Connor, always make sure you've got a good back-up plan." Richard shared that line with Susan during one of their many arguments. She didn't appreciate it.

Richard rarely had a back-up plan, and he had long since tired of the waiting game he had to play when dealing with

Susan, especially since she was the first to note his tardiness if he showed up the standard 10 minutes late.

As an object lesson, Richard would occasionally show up 10-15 minutes late on purpose, in the hopes that she would make an issue of it so that he could blast her for his hour-long wait three days earlier.

The resentment had built to such a point that he found himself spending more time fantasizing about strangling her than making love to her—and it had been over a month since he'd done that. Things were definitely not going well, and sitting and waiting tonight wasn't helping the situation. At 9:45 p.m. the phone rang.

"Hello," he said quietly.

"Richard, where are you?" Susan shouted into the phone. He could tell she was downtown.

"You know where I am. The question is where are you?" he responded.

"I'm downtown. Why didn't you come down and meet me?" she said.

"Because I'm waiting for you here," he said, raising his voice. "You made such a big deal about being ready at 8 o'clock, you said you'd leave if I wasn't ready. Well, it's 9:45 now and where the hell are *you*?"

"I said if I wasn't there by eight, I'd meet you downtown, because I wanted to catch that band."

"I know you wanted to catch that band. So did I. But you distinctly told me that you'd come over and pick me up at eight. Not this 'maybe, maybe not' shit."

"Richard, I remember what I said..."

"No you don't," he interrupted. "And besides, if we were supposed to meet downtown, don't you think we would have set up a meeting spot? Not that you'd get that right, either."

"There's one stage that's set up downtown. Where the hell else would I be?"

"You don't want me to answer that," he said in the most sinister of tones.

"Look, I'm not in the mood to argue," she said. "Do you want to see me tonight or not."

He paused for a few seconds to consider the offer. Love and hate were burning in his mind and body. She didn't apologize for fucking up. She didn't even admit she did anything wrong. It was driving him nuts. Yet, if he stayed home, he would have no avenue to release his anger. And if he got laid, then all might be forgiven and forgotten—for a while, anyway.

"Yeah, I want to see you," he said in a defeated voice.

"Good, 'cause I want to see you," she said a sexy tone. "Now, why don't you come down to The Pub. We'll have some wine, listen to some tunes, and have a good time."

"I'll be down there in a bit," he said.

He hung up the phone and shouted "F-U-U-C-C-K" at the top of his lungs. He took a few deep breaths to calm himself down, chugged the half can of beer in his hand, threw it down, and marched outside to his bike.

He took a longer route to The Pub because he wanted to be as calm as possible when he saw her. He was afraid if he went directly there, he might start yelling immediately.

When he got to The Pub, he was calm and had a nice buzz from the four beers he drank on the couch. He walked in and saw Susan sitting at the bar. They made eye contact and she gave him that look that used to make him melt. Now that same look was having trouble getting through the ice wall he'd been building. She'd have to do more than just look to break through this time.

"Hey babe," she said. "You want a beer?"

He nodded his approval and she had the bartender bring a glass of wine and a pint of The Pub's homemade amber ale that Richard loved. She started talking about the show downtown.

"I don't want to hear about the fucking show," he said evenly. "It brings back memories of me on a couch waiting for you to show up."

She talked about other things, but he just stared straight ahead, drank his beer, and tuned her out. Thoughts of love and hate swarmed around his head again. When she asked him a question, he would give a one word answer.

She tried to loosen him up, with some success. After a half-hour, Richard was stringing together sentences. He still wasn't his usual convivial self, though.

Richard hailed the bartender for another round when he heard some women shout Susan's name. He turned around and saw three young women of the counter-culture persuasion sitting at a table in the corner. Susan responded to them with a "Hey," and told Richard she'd be right back. He asked her if she wanted another glass of Chardonnay, to which she responded with a positive nod.

When he got the drinks he turned around and leaned back against the bar to survey the tavern. He sipped his beer slowly, keeping a close watch on his drinking. He'd already had more than enough for one night, and he didn't want his anger toward Susan to result in a hangover in the morning.

He tried to take his mind off of that anger by listening to the soft jazz being played by the band the bar had hired. When the band stopped for a break, he looked down at his watch and nearly 30 minutes had passed since Susan went over to talk to her friends. She was still there, yapping away.

The band came back on stage and played another set, their final of the evening, and called it a night. Richard looked at his watch and saw that it was midnight. Susan had been talking to the hippies for an hour and 15 minutes.

He looked next to him and saw his empty beer mug next to her full glass of wine. He'd had enough. He drank the glass of wine in one gulp and walked out.

When he got home, he filled a cup with ice water to rehydrate a little before he went to bed, so he wouldn't be hung over in the morning. He went out on the porch and began to contemplate the fact that it was at last truly over between them.

To his surprise, the feeling that filled up inside him was not one of sadness or anger, but one of relief. He had finally freed himself of the chain she'd held around his heart. He could now get on with his life—or so he thought.

As he expected, she rode up a few minutes later.

"Where'd you go?" she asked.

"I left," he said. "I don't like sitting by myself at a bar. I can sit by myself at home and have more peace and quiet."

"Well, what are you doing now?"

"I'm going to sleep."

"But I didn't get to spend any time with you," she said in a pathetic tone.

"That's because you fucked me over twice tonight."

"You left. How do you figure I fucked you over?"

"Susan, when you invite me out, it's with the understanding that we'll be spending the majority of the evening together. I don't mind you talking to friends, but to leave me sitting alone at the bar for over an hour is ridiculous."

"I'm sorry, I hadn't seen them in a long time. Besides, you knew I was with you."

"That's the point," he said raising his voice slightly. "You weren't with me. You were with them. You know, it's not rude to say you're with someone else and you'll catch up with them some other time. It is rude, however, to invite me out and then leave me hanging at the bar like some loser. Then again, being rude to me doesn't seem to faze you."

"Aw babe, I'm sorry. If I'd known you were gonna take it this way, I wouldn't have done it."

"Yeah, you would've. You don't even realize you're doing anything wrong because you take me for granted."

"No, I definitely do not."

"Yeah, you do. You just don't realize it," he said and paused to gather his thoughts. "Look Susan, I'm sick of this whole thing. The miscommunications. The arguments. The lack of input I get. The sexual frustration. The bullshit. I'm tired of it. I'm tired of wondering how late you're gonna be when we make plans. I'm tired of wondering whether or not you're with me when we go out. I know you don't do these things to piss me off on purpose, Susan. You're a good person, and you don't mean anyone harm—especially me. But I just can't take it anymore. Your unpredictability has become way too predictable.

"Remember my response when you said, 'I hope this relationship doesn't end in a negative way?'" Richard paused only to catch his breath. He didn't want to give her a chance to speak and ruin his response to his own question. "I told you that no relationship can end negatively if you learn something from it and are wiser for the experience.

"Well, I'm going to tell you the most important lesson I've learned from this relationship, Susan. It's that it doesn't pay to be a pushover, no matter how much you love someone. As soon as you bend over backwards a little for someone, they want you to bend just a little bit more. And they'll keep bending you until your back is broken and your face is in the dirt and you have nothing to show for it. That's why the meek inherit the earth, Susan. They don't have anything else but heartache from being taken advantage of."

"I didn't take advantage of you," she cried.

"The hell you didn't," he screamed at the top of his lungs.

"I was upfront and honest with you about how I felt the whole time," she screamed back.

"The hell you were," he said in a softer voice, attempting to control his anger. "You knew how I felt all along. You knew what I wanted. And you knew that it wasn't what you wanted.

But instead of sticking to your rules, you tore me apart. You allowed me to stay close because it felt good on most days. And on that one day every four or five weeks when you got claustrophobic, you threw out the stiff arm and reminded me of the ground rules, which were forgotten at your convenience. You were honest, all right. You just didn't know what you wanted. I did, and I've been paying the price for it."

"What did you want me to do, Richard? Would you rather have had me tell you to fuck off and die?"

"Yes, Susan. Believe it or not, I would have preferred it. I'll take the quick, sharp pain over the slow, dull, lingering pain any day. And that's exactly what this relationship has turned into for me."

"I don't understand why we just can't be friends?"

"First of all, we've always been closer than friends," Richard responded.

"You can't get any closer than friends."

"That's weak, Susan," he said in disgust. "I don't have sex with people whom I consider my friends. And if you do, your notion of friendship is screwed up."

"Fuck you," she shouted.

"And besides," he continued, ignoring the insult in order to get his point across, "you knew how I felt about being friends with you. My romantic feelings for you are way too strong to sustain a legitimate friendship. I told you when this whole thing started that you wouldn't be at my wedding unless you were the bride. And it's pretty obvious that no matter what I do, you're not going to be my bride."

"So what are you saying? Is that it?"

"Susan, I'm not like your past boyfriends. I like to keep my life in order and tie up all the loose ends. I've always felt that this relationship would either go up or out. I was hoping that it would go up. But I can see now what you've been saying all along; that as lovers we just don't get along, and that even if we got married we'd end up killing each other."

"That doesn't mean we can't be friends."

"For me it does," he said in a calm, cold tone. "As your friend, all I'll want is more. And I refuse to subject myself to the pain of having you around and yet not being able to have you."

"So that's it? I can't see you any more?" she asked and started to cry.

"Nope," he said, watching her tears begin to flow. He didn't feel bad about seeing her suffer, after all of the suffering he'd been through. It was going just as he promised her, and vowed to himself during times of intense anger. She controlled the relationship while it was alive, but he would ultimately decide when and how it would end. He'd done that now, and it felt good to be the one laying down the ground rules for a change.

"Can I at least send you postcards?"

"Nope," he said, staring at the ground, not wanting to make eye contact and show the sadistic pleasure he was getting from seeing her upset.

"Well, I guess there's nothing more to say except good-bye," she said.

"So long, Susan."

Richard turned and went inside. Before his rear hit the couch, his pleasure from turning Susan away had turned into an overpowering feeling of depressing loneliness. "What did I do?" he asked himself. Those were the last words that escaped his mouth for the next couple of days.

The Couch Weekend

During that weekend Richard didn't eat, sleep or leave the couch except to go to the bathroom. Most of that time was spent staring at the ceiling, in what doctors would later call a "complete clinical depression."

The loneliness that he felt Friday night had progressed on Saturday to a feeling of total hopelessness.

His relationship with Susan had been the oasis in his desert of despair. She had the ability to take him away from the stress of Devlin's missions, if only for a little while. Now that oasis was dry and there was no buffer between his fragile body and this mountain of expectation that he had to climb.

His life was empty. No more school. No more girlfriend. Nothing to take his mind off the mission. Nothing to do now except climb the mountain. All through the relationship, he'd convinced himself that it would end "on his terms." Now that it had, he realized how much he needed her. She'd become an integral part of his life—and he understood only now that it was a part he couldn't live without.

By Sunday he was deeply entrenched on the couch. He began to hallucinate that his soul was separating from his body and sinking below the couch. He could see himself lying pathetically on the couch from a grave's view—six feet under.

In that state, he felt he had no control over his body. His physical self could just get up and walk away and his soul would have no say in the matter because it was stuck in the bowels of the couch. He believed during that separation of mind and body—which only lasted a few hours—that if his body's eyes shut, he would be dead. He looked on, not in fear, but rather in curiosity.

One reason that he wasn't alarmed at what was happening, was that he'd had recurring dreams that were similar to what he was feeling. During his third year in college, he went on a drinking binge that lasted a week. When he came out of it, he felt deathly ill. The doctors at the student infirmary had to dope him up with codeine just so they could run tests to see what was wrong with him. They feared the worst—spinal meningitis. But after numerous tests, they figured out that his low white cell count was not caused by a serious infection or virus. It was created by too much drinking and by running without sufficient sleeping and eating.

While under the codeine trance, Richard hallucinated that he was leaving his body and going down below the bed he was lying on. In the nights that followed, Richard had numerous recurring nightmares that he was leaving his body and descending. He never knew where he was going and he never got there. But the thought of going down rather than up didn't please him in the least.

Richard had entered therapy soon afterward. During one session, he reluctantly told his psychiatrist about the nightmare. He didn't have a whole lot of faith in the psychiatric profession, but he liked what the therapist told him.

"First of all, Richard. Let me be the first to assure you that you're not going to Hell," Dr. Galakawitz said. "This dream of yours is a self-image thing. You see your life going down the tubes, and it manifests itself in this dream. Once you start to feel better about yourself, the dream will stop."

Richard spent that summer building a wood deck in the backyard of his parents' house. He did some running and made sure to stay alcohol-free. By the time the deck was completed, the dream disappeared and never returned.

While the similarity of that recurring dream to his current situation on the couch startled him a little, he definitely noted a difference. His current separation of body and mind felt much more real.

In his dreams he could vividly remember sinking, yet other details were sketchy. In this current depression-induced hallucination, all his senses were heightened. He could smell the exhaust from cars that passed on the street. He could see the tiny moth hanging on the screen door. He could taste the clamminess that pervaded his mouth from days without food or drink. He could hear the drip from the faucet at the kitchen sink. He could feel the threads of the couch through his T-shirt—even though his view was from below the couch. This was all so similar to what he'd experienced before, yet his heightened physical awareness made it so real.

Familiarity with the process was definitely one factor that kept him from panicking. Another was that he wasn't afraid of death. Death used to scare Richard. But the thought of his end didn't disturb him anymore. Neither did the thought of Heaven or Hell. As he was looking from below his body rather than from above, he wondered if his soul would continue to descend, perhaps into Hell.

Growing up in the Jewish faith, he had never been preached to about hellfire and damnation. Surely, bad people paid for their sins. But the fiery underworld ruled by Satan was a Christian concept. In Judaism, Heaven was like a university: if you were good, you were accepted, if you were bad, you were rejected. Of course, if you were rejected, there was no other Heaven you could apply to, so it was kind of important to be good.

Growing up in America had a greater impact on him than his religion, though. And in a country where every public school child is exposed to Christian beliefs, he had gained a healthy respect for Hell—even though his religion didn't clue him into the idea of that horrific hereafter.

He looked up at himself, through the couch, waiting to see what would occur. Life or death—which would it be. Which would his body choose?

Slowly, his soul began to rise up through the couch and merge with his body again. He blinked a few times just to confirm that he had control over his physical self. He was relieved to be at one with himself again.

Richard tried to force positive thoughts into his head. But as he lay on the couch, he thought about his entire life being reduced to one dimension—running—and he felt himself detached from all emotion.

"What am I," he began to ask himself, "if I'm only this one thing?" The answer came to him quickly: "If the only thing I have to contribute to this world is my running, then I have failed in life."

He considered that if he lost a race, he was a failure by everyone's standard. But by being reduced to this one dimension, he was a failure by his own standard.

These negative thoughts of failure ran through Richard's head like a broken record. The sentence that summed it all up, and ran through his head, was: "I don't want to live my life like this any more." By the end of the day that sentence had been reduced to: "I don't want to live my life any more."

When Richard got up, changed and went to practice Monday afternoon, that sense of loneliness and hopelessness he felt throughout the weekend had vanished. It was replaced by a sense of purpose and vitality. He no longer felt burnt out by the heat, the workouts, the races and the expectations. He understood his mission clearly now. It was no longer a question of what place he needed to finish at the SECs, NCAAs, and Olympic Trials. Places no longer mattered. That pressure had been removed. Now the goal was to just run and finish each race so he could move on to the next step and eventually complete the final part of the mission and make peace with himself.

Although he hadn't eaten in three days, he felt fresh on his easy five-miler with Mad Dog. He went home and made a big pot of baked ziti and devoured over half of it. The feeding frenzy disagreed with his stomach, which hadn't seen so much as a drop of water since Friday. But he felt OK again after a visit to the can and a couple of Rolaids.

The next day was a scorcher, 90-plus degrees with over 90 percent humidity. Devlin called practice for 5:30 p.m. instead of 3 p.m. to prevent his runners from having more taken out of them than was needed. It mattered little, though. By the time the distance crew started their workout it was still in the high-80's with the same amount of humidity. And since the workout was so late, the trainers had taken in the water cooler.

Other distance runners complained about the conditions.

None of it affected Richard. He went out and attacked the six repeat 800s, running the last one in 2:01, and blowing away Mad Dog and Anthony. Devlin was pumped after watching him devour the workout, but Richard could care less what Devlin thought.

"Rickey-boy, you're gonna tear 'em up," Devlin said.

"I just want to complete the mission," Richard said quietly and unenthusiastically.

Devlin was starting to worry. He couldn't get Richard to say a sentence anymore that didn't contain the word "mission." But he didn't want to disrupt an elite athlete's mindset, especially one he didn't understand. He figured it was just some psych-up technique Richard was using to get ready for the three big meets coming up. "Crazy distance runners," Devlin would say.

One Step Closer

Going into the SEC Outdoor Championships in Starkville, Mississippi, Richard had all the demeanor of a man going out to mow his lawn. He just didn't care any more. It was a job, not an adventure.

But if his weekend on the couch had drained him, it certainly had its good side. There was no sign whatsoever of any of his pre-SEC rituals. No loss of sleep or appetite. No anxiety. No fear of losing. If he stayed up late it was because he didn't want to sleep, not because he couldn't sleep. Over the course of one weekend, Richard had become the complete antithesis of himself. He was emotionally detached and uncommunicative the entire time he was in Starkville.

Friday, the first day of the meet, was a hot one even by Mississippi late-May standards: 92 degrees with 90 percent humidity. Richard's first race, the 3000-meter steeplechase, was at 3 p.m.—the hottest part of the day. Because of the heat, he didn't need much of a warm-up. He ran 10 minutes around the football practice fields adjacent to the track, and then stretched in the shade.

While he stretched, he watched some of his competitors from Arkansas run as much as 20 minutes in full sweatsuits. Richard, who was wearing a T-shirt and his racing shorts, loved it. Go ahead, he thought. Get a nice sweat worked up underneath all those clothes. You'll be worn out before the race even starts.

Richard took a few practice runs over a hurdle that was set up on the practice field, and then went to the starting line with the other steeplers. On the starting line, Richard was amused at the pre-race tension on the faces of the other runners. That used to be me, he thought. But now I'm free of all that... Thank God!

The gun went off and Richard moved to the front of the pack immediately. Richard often liked to lead in order to set the tempo. He especially liked to lead in the steeplechase because he was not a confident hurdler. Richard always feared that another runner would block his view and cause him to smash into one of the four 75-lb. barriers. He'd seen it happen once before, and it was the first thing on his mind every time he lined up for the steeplechase. By leading, he was able to see the hurdle clearly without having to peer over someone's shoulder.

Richard led the first three laps and felt heavy, despite the relatively slow pace. He told himself that he felt sluggish because of the heat, and that everyone in the race felt sluggish too.

That theory was blown out of the water when he was passed by six runners on the fourth lap—four of whom were Arkansas athletes.

Richard was struggling to hang on to the lead pack. Since his great workout following the weekend on the couch, he'd gone into a slow decline. Too many hard workouts and races in the heat had drained him. He'd run four steeples leading to up the SEC Championships. In the first one, back in April, he ran 8:38.8, which broke Johnny's school record and qualified him for the U.S. Olympic Trials. He'd run progressively slower since then, running an abysmal 9:02 in a meaningless meet in Arboretum one week after his couch retreat.

When the bell rang signifying the last lap of the race, Richard was in seventh place, and five seconds in back of the leader. Just when he thought it was over, his brain shut off and he started moving forward.

With his brain temporarily disconnected, he ran aggressively, attacking and hurdling each barrier as he'd never done before. As he reached the barrier coming off the first curve, he passed three runners to move into fourth place. Over the barrier on the backstretch he passed two more to move into second place. And as he rounded the final curve and approached the water jump, he drew even with the leader, Joe Hall of Auburn.

Making up five seconds in 250 meters had taken a lot out of Richard, who didn't think he'd had a whole lot in the gas tank to begin with. As they sprinted down the homestretch, Joe took the lead and started to pull away.

Joe Hall was a better hurdler than Richard, and had also run a four-minute mile—two seconds faster than Richard's best time. And while Joe seemed to have all the advantages as the two sprinted towards the finish line, Richard had one key factor in his favor: he'd never lost to Joe in anything.

So as Richard struggled to hang on to his apparently superior competitor, he eyed the last barrier on the homestretch — just 50 meters from the finish line. About 15 meters before that last barrier, Joe looked up to see where his rival lurked. When Joe looked back, the barrier was too close to judge and he was forced to stutter step, going straight up and over the barrier and losing all the momentum he'd built up in his sprint. As he came down over the barrier, he watched out the corner of his eye as Richard sailed smoothly over it and past him.

The last 50 meters both athletes put their heads down and went into an all-out sprint. Richard had the momentum from the last barrier and Joe, despite making up some ground, was never able to recover. Richard won by two tenths in 8:48.4.

"You got me again, you son of a bitch," Joe said as the two exhausted runners embraced after the race.

Richard, normally emotional after a big win, was mentally absent. Like the man mowing his lawn, his body had done the work—the brain was disengaged.

Two hours later, Richard and Joe were lined up against each other in the semifinals of the 1500. While warming up, they admitted to each other that the mid-afternoon Mississippi heat had taken a lot out of them in the first race.

Half a mile into the 1500, a race that's 107 meters short of a mile, Richard could see that the steeplechase had exacted a greater toll on his body than on Joe's. Joe won the heat in 3:46, and he looked good doing it. Richard finished fifth in 3:50.8 and looked crappy and beat up.

The fact that Joe won the heat was immaterial. Also immaterial was the fact that Richard made the final by passing four runners in the homestretch and had the slowest qualifying time among the 12 finalists. All that mattered was that both had made Saturday afternoon's final and both would have to face the Canadian Hines and the Irishman Rourke of Arkansas.

Devlin held a team meeting at the hotel that night to discuss the first day's events. He started off by congratulating Richard on his steeple victory and all the "heart he showed in gutting out a tough 1500."

"If everyone shows that kind of heart tomorrow, we got a good shot to beat Arkansas," Devlin said.

Richard received a round of applause from the team, all of whom were packed into Devlin's hotel room. A smile broke out on his face, but not from the embarrassment of the ovation. He thought to himself, What a joke! They think I did this for them. That I took one for the team. They haven't figured it out yet. They think I'm still a part of them. They think I still give a shit whether we win or lose this meet. I barely give a shit whether I win or lose. I'll complete my mission regardless.

Devlin went on to congratulate Mad Dog, who'd beaten all six Arkansas entries in the 10,000, finishing second behind Johnson. Devlin went over some other instructions for the next day and gave a poor excuse for a motivational speech. Richard stood by the door tuning him out and was the first one to leave when the meeting was over.

Richard heard Devlin calling out to him as he walked away. He ignored him just as he'd been doing for weeks. He walked across the street to the Waffle House, the only restaurant within walking distance of the hotel, and ate dinner alone.

While bending over a western omelet with hash browns, cheese grits and toast, he made one small admission to himself. He actually enjoyed his successful day. But winning the steeple and qualifying for the 1500 final was not what tickled him. In his moment of triumph, the thing he was enjoying most was the cold shoulder he was giving his coach; which was just the way Devlin treated him in his moments of disappointment. While Devlin was the head coach, it was common knowledge that he only coached the distance runners. So when one of his boys did well, he loved to be around to experience the joys of victory; just as he hated to be around when things went awry (God forbid someone see him with an FIT distance runner who ran poorly). With all of his success, Richard figured his cold shoulder was probably killing Devlin that night.

He got back to his room and saw the message light blinking on his telephone. He ignored it and went straight to bed.

Richard slept for eight hours without even waking to go to the bathroom—a rarity. He lay in bed until 9 a.m. when he decided that a three-mile run was necessary to determine the severity of the previous day's damage.

He strapped on his shoes and went out for a jog. The results were not positive. He was sore in every muscle area he thought he could be, and a few he didn't even think existed.

He didn't panic, though. He'd been through pain like this before. This was, after all, his 12th SEC championship meet in five years.

After breakfast at the Waffle House, he went to the trainer's room and got a massage and a large dosage of Ibuprofen to help deaden the pain. When he hopped on the bus a few hours later, he was feeling fine.

Richard spent most of the day under the shade of the big tent, drinking water by himself. When a teammate would come over and make an attempt to converse, Richard would give one or two word answers. The teammate would get bored quickly and leave. He heard someone come up behind him and sit down. He looked to his right and it was Devlin.

Richard had no desire to talk to anyone, especially his coach. But he didn't have the desire to move either. So he stayed.

"So you wanna tell me what the fuck is up with you these past few weeks?" Devlin asked.

Richard found Devlin's direct line of questioning to be incredibly humorous. He stared at the ground and said nothing to avoid laughing in Devlin's face. After a few seconds of silence, Devlin went on.

"I can't tell if you're just the most intense athlete I've ever seen, or if you've gone off the deep end. I'm not sure whether to be jacked up about your attitude or concerned."

"Coach, I'm just doing my job, trying to complete the mission," Richard finally responded.

"That's another thing," Devlin said. "You know, when you came into my office back in August and asked me what your mission was, I thought that making your goals a mission was a good idea. Especially since you had trouble in the past keeping focused on those goals. But lately you've been obsessed with it, and it's starting to piss me off. You used to be the most friendly, talkative guy on the team. You were the emotion of the team. Everyone liked you and wanted you to do well. Now that you're kickin' ass, you've lost your personality. Guys on the team come up to me and say, 'What's up with Dick?' You don't talk, or smile, or laugh anymore. I'm glad that you're running well, and I want you to complete your mission, but not if the cost is your sanity—which I've started to question over the past few weeks."

After listening to Devlin's speech, Richard was tempted to say, "You weren't so concerned for my sanity when you roasted me in front of the whole team after I ran like shit at NCAA Indoors." But he didn't. He just wasn't in the mood to argue.

"I don't know what to tell you, Devlin. I'm worn out. I don't want to talk. I don't want to laugh. I just want to run so I can get this whole thing over with. I got the rest of this meet, the NCAAs, the Olympic Trials. When that's over, you can put me in a box—I'm finished forever."

"What the fuck has gotten into you?" Devlin said, clearly puzzled. "I've never seen someone's personality change in such a short period of time."

"Listen, Frank," Richard said, addressing Devlin by his first name for the first time. "I really like sitting here in the shade by the water cooler. It's relaxing. But if you're gonna badger me about something that's none of your damn business, I'm gonna be forced to move. So what's it gonna be?"

Devlin sat there in shock with his mouth open. Not only did an athlete call him by his first name —which was a huge no-no—but the cold, emotionless tone in which Richard said those words was one that Devlin had never heard from him before. After fully taking in what had just taken place, Devlin got up and left without saying another word.

Richard felt as bad on his warm-up jog as he did on the morning run. That was not a good sign. The 1500 was a short race, so he would have no time to get his legs warmed up during the race like he would in the 5000. His legs had to be ready from the starting gun, otherwise he would be left in the dust.

When the gun sounded, his worst fears came true. Four Arkansas runners burst out with an opening sprint. Richard was a full three seconds behind after half a lap. His legs ached and there seemed to be little hope of him placing anywhere but last.

But where the old Richard would begin to feel sorry for himself during a disappointing performance, the new Richard kept calm and kept his head. With two laps to go, there was a pack of ten runners up front and a pack of two —which included Richard—about five seconds back. He knew that all ten wouldn't hold on to the front pack for the last two laps. So he made it his job to catch as much roadkill from the front group as possible.

With one lap to go, Richard had picked off only one from the front group. His legs were feeling better, though, and he sensed that he had more left than anyone up front. It was just a question of how much more. Richard began the final lap by picking up the pace gradually. He couldn't hold a sprint for 400 meters even when he was fresh. Therefore, he would need to build up to top speed slowly. On the backstretch he approached two roadkills and passed them quickly. Passing them gave him a certain momentum and incentive. He knew he was starting to move fast.

He passed two more as he entered the final curve. He looked up to see if he had a shot to catch anyone else. Rourke and Hines of Arkansas were running away with the race. He had no chance to catch them. But there was a pack of three that he thought he might be able to catch.

He came off the curve like a slingshot and set his sights on the three runners who were definitely coming back to him.

Richard kept his eyes open as he shifted into fifth gear. Where did this strength and power come from? he thought. He moved into the inside half of the first lane. He wouldn't be able to pass them if he had to swing out into the third lane to do it. But if the runner on the inside happened to move out just a bit, he could slide in on the inside and pass them all.

With less than 50 meters to go, he had made up all the ground on the threesome, who were running abreast. He waited what seemed to be an eternity for an opening. And when the middle runner drifted out just a bit, Richard burst through the three-man wall and leaned hard at the line to take third in 3:46.4, just a tenth of a second ahead of Joe Hall.

As he walked slowly off the track after the incredible comeback, the first thought that came to Richard's mind was: one step closer to the end.

Two hours later he lined up for the 5000. The 5K at the SEC Outdoor Championships was like a cross country race. Every team lined up four or five runners—or seven in the case of Arkansas—for the final distance event of the day. Milers, 5Kers,

10Kers, steeplechasers, and even a few 800-meter runners. It would be a survival of the fittest.

With 30-40 runners at the starting line, getting into a good position at the start was important. So when the gun went off, Richard threw a few elbows and sprinted out to the lead.

After the first lap, Richard settled into sixth place behind Team Arkansas. Under most circumstances Richard liked to lead a race to establish his tempo. But it took a lot of energy to lead a race, and energy was something that Richard did not have a lot of. The plan was simple: Stay near the leaders, then kick like an angry mule on the last lap. He figured if he could conserve enough energy on the first ten laps, he could pass a lot of people over the last $2^1/_2$ laps. With so many Arkansas runners, plus Johnson—who'd only run one race to his three—he could maybe take a respectable fourth or fifth.

Richard felt sluggish during the first mile, which he went through in 4:31, but like all his races that weekend, he began to feel better as the race progressed. And after two miles, he caught a second wind for the umpteenth time that weekend.

He looked up and saw that the lead group had only about a four-second lead on him. Two laps later, he caught the lead pack and felt ready to go with anyone who wanted to try breaking away over the last $2^1/_2$ laps.

There's usually a build-up in the last few laps of a distance race that culminates in an all-out sprint to the finish. With $1^1/_2$ laps remaining, Richard sensed none of that build-up. There was no nervous switching of positions by the athletes, and the pace remained as it was during the first 11 laps—a consistent 67-68 seconds a lap. It was as if the other guys were sleepwalking. Could they possibly be more tired than he? Had the long meet taken its toll on everyone? The thought that juggernauts like Terry Johnson and David Allen could actually get tired seemed preposterous. But as the front pack rounded the curve with just over a lap remaining, no one was poised to make a move. So Richard did.

With 500 meters ($1^1/_4$ laps) remaining, Richard flashed past the six other runners in the lead pack. Like the 1500, Richard picked up the pace continuously throughout the first half of the final lap, waiting for the all-out sprint. With 200 meters left, he looked over his shoulder to see where the competition was. They weren't there!

Richard stared over his shoulder in shock and almost

tripped over the inside railing. He figured he must have put three seconds on the lead pack in just over half a lap. He cruised the last 200 meters and won easily in 13:58.78—a time fast enough to qualify him for the NCAA championships in the 5000.

After he crossed the finish line he shook his head and wondered, "Am I really that good, or did they just give me that race?"

His curiosity was heightened when he saw Johnson come across the line in second place. Johnson looked barely out of breath. Could it be possible that Johnson let him win? Richard, puzzled, caught up with Johnson on his cool-down jog and asked him point blank.

"What the hell happened?" Richard asked.

"I thought I had it won until you snuck up on me, you son of a bitch," Terry chuckled. "I was gonna wait until about 400-to-go to start picking it up, but you already had over a second on me by that point. When I saw that, I kind of gave up and jogged it in. I figured our team had no chance of winning anyway, so why bust my balls? Might as well save it for a more important day."

Richard was not surprised to hear that Terry didn't go all-out to catch him, as *he* most assuredly would have. He knew Terry had the right philosophy toward his running career—don't kill yourself in the smaller meets with the big ones only a few weeks away. And compared to the Olympic Trials, the SEC Championship was minuscule.

Devlin would probably consider Johnson's attitude to be wimping out. "If you don't race to win every time out, then you ain't a very competitive person," he would say.

Nothing could be further from the truth when talking about Johnson. Richard knew that Johnson's "Gambler" philosophy—knowing when to hold 'em and when to fold 'em—would probably land him a spot on the only team that matters in the sport of track and field—the Olympic team. That kind of competitive restraint was something neither Richard nor Devlin knew anything about.

Payback

When the plane landed in Arboretum Monday afternoon,

Richard hopped in his car and took off toward home. He hit the bed seconds after he opened the door. He slept for four hours, woke up to eat, and then slept another eight, waking only twice because of leg cramps.

He awoke for good at 8 a.m. when the phone rang. He answered and recognized Devlin's voice.

"Rickey-boy, get your ass up to my office," Devlin commanded. "We need to talk about something."

Richard put on shorts, a T-shirt, and a pair of sandals and rode up to school. He didn't want to see Devlin, but Devlin was still the coach. So 20 minutes after the coach called, a sleepy-eyed Richard was in Devlin's office.

Devlin threw a copy of the local newspaper at Richard as he sunk into the soft sofa by the door. Richard picked it up and saw a picture of himself on the front page. It showed him during the last lap of the SEC steeplechase as he came out of the water pit. An ironic smile broke on his face as he read the headline: "FIT Runner on a Mission."

The article read:

> Starkville, Miss—Although the FIT Men's Track Team finished a disappointing second place in this weekend's SEC Outdoor Championship—25 points behind Arkansas—no one could say Richard Dubin contributed to the disappointment.
>
> Dubin was a double winner in the 3000-meter steeplechase and the 5000-meter run. The senior also finished third in the 1500.
>
> In all, Dubin scored 26 of his team's 97 points and was named the meet MVP—an award that hasn't been given to a distance runner in 14 years.
>
> "This meet and the NCAA meet [next week in Austin, Texas] is all just a build-up to Olympic Trials," Dubin said. "The ultimate goal of every runner is to make the Olympic team. I'm no different." The Trials will be held June 17-30 in New Orleans.

The article went on to quote Devlin, who talked about what a "fine, hard-working, young man" Richard was. Devlin was also quoted as saying, "Hard work and good coaching usually lead to successful results."

Richard shook his head in disgust as he read Devlin's quote, but he smiled when he read the ending:

> "I'm on a mission right now," Dubin says. "For better or worse, that mission will end in New Orleans."

"So what do you think, Rickey-boy?" Devlin said, expecting an enthusiastic answer.

"I don't give a shit," Richard said.

"The hell you don't," Devlin said, clearly perturbed. "Everyone takes pride in their accomplishments."

"I do, too," he rebutted. "I just care very little anymore about SEC's or NCAA's. I've grown tired of beating the shit out of my body to score points for your championships. It doesn't motivate me anymore. I'd quit, except I made a commitment. That commitment ends after the next meet. Then I'm done with you."

"What are you saying? You gonna tank it and save yourself for the Trials?" Devlin asked.

"Not at all," Richard responded quickly. "I'll give it all I've got. That's all I know how to do, Devlin. Just because I don't want to run the meet, doesn't mean I won't try my hardest once the gun goes off. I'm a competitive guy. I want to win everything I run—even the races I don't want to run."

"Well, since you don't care about the fucking meet, I suppose you don't care what you run," said an exasperated Devlin.

"Put me in whatever you want. I don't care."

"Fine. I'll enter you in the 5K and the steeplechase. How's that?" Devlin said.

"If that's what you want me to run, Coach, that's what I'll run," Richard said calmly, as he got up and moved toward the door. "I want to let you in on a little secret that you haven't seemed to catch on to after five years. You never need to doubt the fact that I'm giving my all in every race. That's just the way I am. All I know is 'Go,' and I never hold back. So the times you've accused me of not trying during a bad race have only led to a general lack of respect for you as my coach. That level of respect is now at a five-year low.

"One other thing," he said. "Ever since I came to this awful place I've been made to feel that I'm not worthy of the scholarship I've received. Every summer when I'd re-sign the scholarship sheet, you'd always remind me of the things I did wrong and how lucky I was to hold on to it. I almost lost it a couple of years ago before I got my mind straight. You made me feel so fucking guilty when I signed the scholarship sheet that year. But every year, even that bad one, I was good enough to keep it.

"I never liked this place, Devlin. Every year I thought about going elsewhere. But I stayed, partly because I thought that leaving would be the equivalent to admitting failure, but more because I had a sense of loyalty to this school and to you. I can see now, that my major failure was in never leaving, and my loyalty to you was a wasted effort. I've been sorry I came to this hellhole since Day One. But I've been worth every fucking penny of scholarship I ever got because I've risen above the lousy coaching I've received."

Richard didn't give Devlin a chance to respond. He closed the door behind him and walked swiftly out of the building, confident that he'd gotten at least some payback for the public humiliation he'd received after the NCAA indoor meet.

At practice that afternoon, Devlin gave out the workout sheet for the week and the itinerary for their trip to Austin the following week. Richard and Mad Dog were the only distance runners to qualify for NCAA's. Therefore, they were the only distance runners doing the workouts that week. Devlin supervised their workouts without saying a word to either of them. He wore the look of a man managing a really bad baseball club; he was angry, distrustful, tired, and ready for the long season to end. That was one department where Devlin and Richard had something in common.

Paroled

When the 12 members of the team who qualified for the NCAA Outdoor Championships boarded the plane to go to Austin on the first Monday in June, Richard was in good spirits. While most of his teammates whined and complained of summer boredom in a college town, especially those who chose not to enroll in summer school, Richard—the recent graduate—spent his free time doing things he'd always wanted to do.

First on his hit list was certain books he wanted to read. Richard was not well-read and always regretted not reading some of the great American novels. He finished *Moby Dick* in four days, *Absalom! Absalom!* in two days, and brought *Catch-22* on the plane with him. He also went skydiving and bungee-jumping about 30 miles south of Aboretum.

Richard planned to use the three weeks between the SEC meet and Olympic Trials wisely. Run a little, plan a little, and spend the rest of the time enjoying himself.

On the plane, everyone looked intense. The school had never brought home an NCAA championship before in any sport. But with 12 athletes competing in ten different events, they were considered one of the favorites.

They'd been in that position before. Richard's sophomore and junior year, the Aggies were favored to win their first championship. False starts, disqualifications, and generally poor performances—as was the case with Richard—cost them the title both years. Richard looked at the tense faces of his teammates and knew this meet—just like indoor season—would be another chapter in the Aggies' Journal of Underachievement at the NCAA Championships.

Richard threw his stuff down and was out the door as soon as the team reached the hotel. He had no idea where he was going, but with his first race on Wednesday, he wasn't about to sit around the hotel and mope for two days. That was the old Richard—the one who feared success almost as much as he dreaded failure. With all that mental baggage now gone and his eyes wide open for the first time in his adult life, he went out to explore and see places he'd never been before.

When the gun sounded Wednesday night for the start of the steeplechase trials, Richard had only one thought in his head, expend as little energy as possible, but above all, make it to Friday's final.

He'd had an interesting two days exploring Austin. He especially liked the downtown area. He made sure, though, that he didn't wear out his racing legs from walking too much. Richard slept ten hours a day to make sure he had enough rest for steeplechases on Wednesday and Friday, as well as 5Ks on Thursday and Saturday.

He was confident. But, as the race progressed, he made no blind assumptions that he would be able to walk into the steeple final. There were many fine athletes—more than the 14 allowed into the final—and he knew he would have to work to make it there.

Although he struggled with his hurdling form and felt heavy-legged throughout the race, he finished fifth in the second of two qualifying heats. That was good enough to advance to Friday night's final.

He felt ready to go for the 5K heat when he woke up Thursday morning. But when the gun went off Thursday night, it was Nightmare at Nationals Part II.

Even though the race went out very slow, Richard still felt terrible. After the group went through the first mile in a pathetic 4:45, everyone picked up the pace drastically. Everyone, that is, but Richard.

Richard spent the last two miles watching helplessly as the leaders extended their lead on him. He crossed the finish line last in his heat in 15:10.

He walked off the track to the athlete's tent to get his gear. On his way, he passed Devlin, who was sitting in the first row of the stands. Devlin's cold stare was saying, "Once again, you're an embarrassment to me at the NCAAs."

Richard stared straight back at him and shrugged. His look and body language said, "What the hell do you expect? This is my sixth race in the past two weeks. If you didn't want to be embarrassed at this meet, you shouldn't have had me run four races a week and a half ago."

Richard didn't fret about the dirty looks from Devlin. He expected those, especially after his speech in Devlin's office the week before. What worried Richard most was that he had another race to run the next day. And Number 7 in the past two weeks was no 1500 or 5000. It was the one with the 28 barriers and seven water jumps. If there was ever a race he wished he could drop out of, it was Friday's steeple final. He knew there was no way out, though. So he just resigned his body to one more beating. He slept long and deep Thursday night and prepared for his last race under Devlin's tyranny.

Coming into Friday's steeple final, Richard took what he referred to as the masochist's point of view, which says: This race is going to hurt, so I might as well enjoy the pain. The approach rarely helped him come race time, except to make the misery more satisfying.

So when he stood at the starting line, Richard was in good spirits, almost reveling in the other competitors' angst and pain. He wanted to do well, but he expected nothing. His body had already given him enough over the previous weeks and he could ask for no more. He would take whatever he could get.

The gun sounded and Richard darted aggressively to the front of the pack and settled in on the leader's shoulder. He stayed there for the first three laps but began to fall off the pace as he did in the 5000. With two laps left in the race, Richard was well back of the leaders, but runners who tried to hold on were beginning to come back to him. He smelled blood and tried to pick up the pace. Amazingly, his body responded. In the last two laps he went from 13th place to eighth, which earned him an All-American award and scored one point for the team.

He walked off the track proud of his effort. More importantly, though, he was done with Devlin.

Back at the athlete's tent, Richard gathered his gear and prepared to go back to the hotel. He turned to leave and bumped straight into Devlin.

"Well, Rickey-boy, what do you have to say for yourself?"

"I say I'm proud of the effort I've put out for you for the past five years. I've done my time and now I've been paroled."

With that, Richard took off his FIT racing singlet, handed it to Devlin, and walked away.

1

Shopping

Richard and Johnny arrived in New Orleans, Saturday afternoon, two days before their race. The Olympic Committee assigned rooms by event. So Richard and Johnny coordinated their travel and hotel plans to avoid being stuck with a competitor they didn't like. When they got to the Hyatt Regency, they threw down their stuff, put on their running shoes, and went out for an easy five miler.

Although Richard had two weeks to recover from the seven races he ran between SECs and NCAAs, he still felt worn down. He knew he had it in him to make the steeplechase final at Olympic Trials. He also knew to expect nothing of himself, especially after his poor performance at NCAAs.

The first round would be Monday night, where they would cut three heats of 12 runners (36), down to two (24) for Wednesday night's semifinal. The top six runners in each of the three heats automatically qualified for the semis; and the top six times among the leftovers would also qualify. Wednesday's semifinal would be purely a race for place—the top seven in each heat, regardless of time, would fill the field of 14 for Friday's final.

After the five-mile run, Richard showered and dressed. He grabbed the $150 in cash he had in his bag beside the bed and walked out the door without saying a word to Johnny.

By asking directions along the way, Richard found his way to the French Quarter. It was about a mile walk from the Hyatt.

Carrying $150 in cash on his person made Richard a bit nervous. He carried the money in the front pocket of his shorts, and kept his hands in his pockets at all times. He didn't want some thief who was feeling frisky to destroy his plans and ruin the mission.

He constantly looked behind him on his trek into the Quarter and decided if a thief held him up at gun or knifepoint, he'd call the criminal's bluff and make a run for it. He figured his chances were pretty good that a small-time thief's aim at a moving target under pressure was poor, and that a thief near the Quarter wouldn't really want to shoot anyway and alert the numerous cops in the vicinity. Besides, he knew he was faster than just about any thief—unless the thief happened to be competing in the Olympic Trials as well.

He wandered the streets of the Quarter at dusk and took in all the sights (mostly bars and topless joints) and smells (mostly urine, stale beer, and vomit). He stopped in at a place on Bourbon Street called Renee's Gun Shop.

"Welcome to Renee's," said the short, solidly-built, 60-something man behind the counter. He chose to put the accent on the first syllable in "Renee," making his name rhyme with "penny." Richard had always heard that name with the second syllable accented. He figured it must be a Cajun thing.

"I'm surprised you're open this late," Richard said using the mild southern accent he'd picked up from his five years in Arboretum. "Most gun shops around where I live aren't open at 6:30."

"We like to work things a little differently here," the man said. "You'll notice we don't have our hours of business posted on the door. We stay open as long as the sun's up."

"I guess that means I don't have a lot of time," Richard said, pointing outside to the setting sun.

"Oh, you'll be all right. The only time I've ever kicked customers out to close shop were on the eight days my children were born. And most of 'em were born in the early afternoon so I was able to come back and open up shop again," he said and burst forth with a good-natured belly laugh.

"Then I take it you're Renee," Richard said, correctly accenting the first syllable.

"At your service for 35 years," he said.

"That's a lot longer than I've been alive," Richard said, and they both laughed.

Richard told Renee that he needed a gun for "personal protection." Renee showed him a series of handguns in his price range.

Richard knew that the state of Louisiana hadn't come around like most other states in instituting a waiting period before buying a gun.

Out of curiosity, he asked Renee's opinion on that issue, Renee responded quickly: "Hell, someone wants to kill a person, ain't no waiting period gonna stop 'em."

As for a national computerization check before a gun can be purchased, he said: "Shoot! They don't need to check the people coming in my store. The criminals don't come in here. Ain't never been a murder weapon traced back to this store in all 35 years I've been in business. The murderers get their guns out on the street. Same place they get their drugs. There are so many guns being sold illegally on the street nowadays. That's where the computer check should be set up."

Richard bought a "slightly used" Smith & Wesson pistol for $125 and a box of 50 .32 caliber shells for $15. Renee also gave him a paper bag to carry the gun and shells back to the hotel. He clutched the bag tightly, not letting it dangle from his hand, for fear that someone might run by and swipe it from him.

When he got back to the hotel, Johnny was not in the room. Richard took advantage of the situation. He took the gun and the ammunition out of the box. He loaded the gun—the way Renee had showed him—and stuffed it in his bag. He took the boxes and bags and discarded them in one of the dumpsters behind the hotel. Richard rubbed his hands clean and went to dinner.

Round One

Richard slept well Sunday night—the night before his first-round race. He got nine hours of sound sleep. He was sleeping and eating like a king in New Orleans, even better than he'd done before the SEC and NCAA meets. Part of it was that he was free of Devlin and his expectations. But there was more to it than that. Richard had totally convinced himself that he would enjoy his last week and not get caught up in the hoopla of an event that used to mean everything to him, but now meant almost nothing.

It was all a game to him now. How far could he go? How far could he exceed the expectations of others. But no matter what, the race was not going to get in the way of him enjoying the experience.

Richard went out after breakfast and walked around the Quarter by himself for a few hours.

He drifted by a vintage clothing store and thought of Susan. He walked in and saw some gowns from the 1920's that were faded, yet still elegant, and some beaded sweaters—all clothes that Susan would wear.

Has it really been a month since our breakup? he asked himself. It all seemed like such a distant memory to him now.

It was nearly noon and Richard didn't want to miss lunch. The meals for the athletes were in a catering hall in the hotel. The food was excellent, and it was all you could eat.

Previously, Richard had eaten with reckless abandon. But as he got on the buffet line, eyeing the prime rib, he reminded himself that he had a race to run that night, and needed to watch what went into his body.

He passed up the prime rib and went instead for the pasta primavera. This wasn't much of a sacrifice, since Richard was an indiscriminate eater and preferred quantity over both quality and choice. With the pasta, he could stuff himself at lunch and feel fine for the race seven hours later. He stayed away from the vegetables because they were gaseous and might cause cramps. He also made sure to treat himself to a small ice cream cone afterward—which he figured would have no effect in seven hours.

He finished the cone as he walked up to his room. He visited the bathroom and then crawled up under the sheets and took a two-hour nap. When he woke up he looked over at the clock. It was nearly 3 p.m.—four hours till race time. He saw Johnny sitting up in bed, reading.

Richard flipped on the TV and watched a stupid movie while he performed his pre-race ritual: pin the race number to the uniform, put the uniform and the racing spikes in the carry bag, put on the underwear, shorts and socks that he would race in, and put on the T-shirt he would warm up in. Apart from that, the only other ritual he had was to drink as much water as he could, and go to the bathroom as often as he needed.

At 5 p.m. he picked up some rolls that the caterers were laying out for dinner, and then hopped on the bus to go to the track. Johnny sat beside him on the bus, but few words were spoken. Johnny was off in a distant land that Richard couldn't reach. If Johnny wanted to talk, he'd say something; otherwise, Richard would leave him alone. This meet meant a lot more to Johnny than it did to him, and Johnny's mental preparation was important.

When they got to the track they went over to the athlete

check-in tent and signed in for their event. They went to the warm-up field, adjacent to the track, where some of the other athletes were sitting and they hung out for a half-hour. Richard chatted with some of his friends who would be running the steeple, including his old rival, Joe Hall. Johnny just lay down on the grass and stared at the sky.

At 6 p.m., Richard, Johnny and a few others went on a three-mile warm-up run. As the group was laughing and joking on the run, Richard noticed Johnny was not a part of the group. Johnny ran ahead and took a quick right turn and left the group. Richard thought about going with him, but decided he was relaxing pleasantly with the group. He figured Johnny wanted to be alone, anyway.

After the warm-up, the group stretched and did some strides. He didn't see Johnny until the group entered the warm-up pen at the track 20 minutes before the first heat of the steeple—in which they were both entered.

All 36 steeplers were packed into the warm-up pen—a four-lane straightaway about 50 meters long. Hurdles were set up in two of the four lanes so the steeplers could practice. Of course, regular hurdles that fall over don't prepare you for the 75-lb. barriers that don't budge, but Richard laced up his spikes and took his token practices anyway.

An official called the first heat over to the tent in the pen and gave the group stick-on hip numbers to wear. Richard was given "1", and Johnny was given "7". They looked at each other and smiled at the numbers they drew. It was the first sign of life from Johnny since they arrived in New Orleans.

Another official lined the first heat up single file and marched them out to the track. The 12 runners were given two minutes to run some strides and take a practice jump or two over the barriers. They were then lined up at the starting line by order of their hip numbers.

It all seemed to be moving too fast, and just as Richard was getting his wits about him, the gun went off. A quick thought went through his head, "I'm running in the Olympic Trials right now." And then his mind went into race mode.

Richard made sure he stayed in the front of the pack for the first few laps to get the best view of the barrier. He didn't want to get passed until the crowd thinned out a little. He wanted to concentrate on every barrier. He didn't care if he stepped on them or hurdled them, as long as he didn't stutter-step. And if

I do stutter, he thought, don't curse yourself for the next 70 meters and screw up the next barrier. . . And for God's sake, DON'T FALL!

Richard led for the first two laps. But the pace he set was slow, and some of the big boys started getting antsy. Fifty meters into the third lap, eight runners swept past him, including Johnny. They picked up the pace and Richard couldn't hang with them. The new front pack opened up a three-second gap on the third lap and extended it to 10 seconds with two laps remaining.

Richard was languishing in 11th place with two laps to go, and looked to be out of the running. But that was when his brain shut off and his pride took over.

Richard began an all-out sprint that didn't stop until the finish line. In those two laps, Richard hurdled every barrier, didn't stutter on any approaches, passed three people, and made up four seconds on the lead pack.

Richard realized none of this. He saw what he did on the replay screen in the Competitor's Room—the area that all the runners are ushered to after their race. Watching closely for place and time, Richard saw that he finished eighth in 8:41. Now he had to wait, count places, and see if his time would get him into the semifinal.

A Fading Memory

After they were released from the Competitor's Room, Johnny and Richard ran their four-mile cool-down from the track back to the hotel.

They made it to the next round. Johnny was fifth in the first heat and qualified automatically by finishing in the top six. He ran 8:34.58—a personal best—and said he felt comfortable. Richard qualified based on time. His 8:41.72 ranked fifth among those who did not finish in the top six in their heat. The guy who ranked seventh—the first man out—ran 8:41.81.

When he saw the times, and how close he was to being eliminated, Richard laughed. "I prayed to the God of Time last night," he told some of his friends in the Competitor's Room.

After a shower, Richard told Johnny he was going to head down to the French Quarter to blow off a little steam. Johnny was not interested. He planned on showering and going right to bed.

Richard noticed something very different about Johnny. He was more serious and focused about his running than Richard had ever seen. He wasn't drinking or partying. It was eerie, he thought. This man that he'd known so well for five years was all of a sudden a completely different person, much like Devlin said *he'd* become after the couch weekend.

Richard had hoped to confide in Johnny some of the thoughts that were going through his mind during the completion of his "mission." Now Richard was afraid to say anything to him. He felt like he didn't know Johnny any more and was no longer comfortable around him.

Richard got dressed and began walking towards the French Quarter. The goal was not to get drunk that night, but just to air out some of his thoughts and reflect on the events of the day.

It was a typically humid night in New Orleans, but with a light, cool breeze that felt good as it ran through his hair. When he reached the Quarter, Richard ducked into one of the less crowded bars along Bourbon Street. He saw Terry Johnson sitting at the bar, drinking alone. Earlier that evening—just before Richard's race—Johnson won the 10,000 meters and made his first Olympic team.

While the "experts" considered his victory a major upset—he'd finished only fifth at the national meet the year before—Richard was not surprised at all. Although Johnson had never won an NCAA title, he hadn't lost to an American in over a year. He was tough, motivated, smart and always prepared. The bigger the race, the more prepared he was.

So Richard wasn't surprised at Johnson's success. But the way he won it *was* a surprise. Johnson had pulled away with 3000m to go and opened an insurmountable 15-second lead that even the fastest finishers couldn't dream of overcoming.

"I suppose congratulations are in order," Richard said as he bellied up at the bar next to Johnson, who smiled, said thanks, and shook Richard's hand.

"So how does it feel?" Richard asked.

"Pretty good. I'm happy," he said in a quiet, almost glum tone that didn't sound at all convincing. Johnson seemed almost disappointed.

"I gotta be honest, Terry. You don't sound like a person who just made his first Olympic Team," Richard said. "In fact, you sound more like the guy who finished fourth."

"No, I'm happy," he said. "It's just that I expected more than I should have out of the whole thing."

Richard gave a puzzled look and Johnson went on to explain.

"Well, you know how it is, Dick. It's like you work so hard for this one thing, with one goal in mind—making The Team. You focus all your energy on it for years. Then when you're coming into the home stretch, you realize that in a few seconds you're gonna achieve that goal, and that dream that you worked so hard for is gonna come true. And for those last few seconds of the race you're on top of the world. You're King of the Mountain. Then the race ends and the moment's over. It's just a memory that fades every second. Now you're not just an Olympian, you're an American Olympian, where anything other than gold is looked upon as second rate. And you're a complete failure if you don't win a medal.

"One thing I'll never forget," he continued, "is that feeling I had right after I crossed the line. I remember the first words I said to myself: 'Is that it?' All that work, and all I can think to say to myself is, 'Is that it?' I mean, I don't know exactly what I expected to feel afterward. I didn't expect to see God at the finish line. But I was hoping for at least a more intense feeling of accomplishment. Something longer-lasting.

"I guess I had my celebration on the home stretch. But now it feels like just another race in a season with more important races yet to come. I just wish the celebration could have lasted longer."

Johnson was not a man of many words. His nickname at Tennessee was "Robo-runner," and he liked to enhance that intimidating image by showing no emotion and saying little. He didn't allow many people to know his feelings, so Richard was surprised by not only by the quantity, but the content of Terry's words. He was shocked that Terry had opened up to him at all.

He showed respect for Johnson's feelings by observing a moment of silence to allow the full effect of his words to sink in. Then Richard spoke: "You remind me of this movie called *The Candidate*. Robert Redford plays a young guy who gets talked into running for the U.S. Senate against the old incumbent, who's held the office for a long time and is the heavy favorite to win again. Well, the last scene in the movie, Redford is sitting in his hotel room. His campaign manager, Peter Boyle, comes into the room to celebrate the fact that he's pulled the upset. But Redford has this long look on his face, kinda like you. Boyle looks at him and says, 'What's wrong? You've won.' He looks at Boyle and says 'What do I do now?'"

A smile broke out on Johnson's face and it was accompanied by a positive nod. They both knew what would happen to Johnson at the Olympics. He, along with the rest of the American distance runners, would be humbled by the Africans and go home with their tails between their legs. Even so, it was an honor that many—including Richard—would give a limb to attain.

The two drank pretty much in silence for another ten minutes. Richard finished his beer and wished Johnson luck at the Games. He got up and walked back to the hotel. Johnny was asleep and so was Richard as soon as he hit the pillow.

Round Two

Richard went through the same routine for his second round race on Wednesday as he did on Monday: sleep, eat, explore the city, eat, sleep, drink lots of water and go to the bathroom often.

While his daily routine was the same—right down to the amount of time he warmed up—the race strategy would be completely different. In round one he could qualify on time if he didn't finish in the top six in his heat. Round two was a race purely for place. The top seven in each heat made the finals. It didn't matter if the eighth place runner in one heat ran faster than the winner of the other. Some runners complained about one heat having better runners than the other. But the two semi-final heats were determined by the performances in the first round. The process was non-prejudicial and didn't play favorites. It was cruel, but fair.

Richard and Johnny were in the same heat again—this time the second. And again, Johnny went off and warmed up by himself, while Richard ran with Joe Hall, who had also survived the first-round cut.

Because the race was just for place and time was not a determining factor, Richard had to rethink his strategy. He had struggled as the leader in the first two laps of his first round race. So when the gun went off, he tucked in on the shoulder of the leader, Mike Cook, the winner of Richard's first-round heat, and concentrated on attacking the barrier on stride. The plan was to save as much energy as he could for the final two laps, which would no doubt require a hellacious finish to make the final.

Running beside Cook was demoralizing for Richard. It wasn't that Cook was such an intimidating runner. In fact, his best times for all events other than the steeplechase were not too much better than Richard's best times. But Cook was a great hurdler. His technique was textbook: approach, glide over and recover. He could only hurdle with one leg—his left—but his depth perception was so good that he never stutter-stepped, even when he was tired or someone was blocking his view. He was a machine; no matter the conditions, he would get over the hurdle smoothly.

Every time they went over a barrier Richard would lose three meters to Cook, even when he attacked and hurdled in stride. With 28 barriers and seven water jumps, that meant a lot of meters for him to make up.

As the race wore on, Richard became more and more fatigued by having to make up ground lost over the barriers. He could tell Cook was comfortable and under control, waiting patiently for the final two laps to explode. Richard wondered if he would have any gas left in the tank for that two-lap sprint to the finish line.

But the good news for Richard was that he didn't have to beat Cook to make the final; he just had to finish seventh out of 12. Surely, he thought to himself, there were five guys back there who were as tired as he was. And if they were that tired, he could take them in a two-lap race. And if he couldn't, he wanted to at least cross the line knowing he gave it everything he had. If this was going to be his last race, he was going to make damn sure he went down swinging.

When Richard and Cook crossed the line with two laps remaining, the crowd that had followed close behind for the entire race began to close in on them. Richard became claustrophobic, but he was too tired to do anything about it.

Cook picked up the pace and left Richard. A group of about nine others, including Johnny, went with him. All of a sudden

Richard was in 11th place again. He didn't panic, though.

Cook continued the gradual pickup and the pack began to spread out a bit. Richard hung on to the back of the pack, and when the bell rang signaling the final lap, he was still within striking distance.

He went by #10 before he went into the first turn and caught up to #9 in the turn. He passed him on the backstretch and began making up ground on #8. Into the final turn he drew even with #8 on the approach to the water jump. Coming off the final turn into the homestretch he blew by him and went into an all-out sprint. The gap to #7 was 15 meters as Richard approached the final barrier. He saw #7 struggle over that barrier as he approached it like gangbusters. Concentrate, he told himself. If you don't hit this last one perfectly, you're through. He lengthened his stride and hurdled it without losing any momentum. He was catching #7, but he wasn't sure if he would have enough track left to pass him. He put his head down but kept his eyes open so he could see in front of him. #7's shoes appeared in his vision with about 40 meters to go. He looked up and saw that #7 was drifting to the outside of the first lane. In a decision that was made purely by instinct, Richard moved to the inside of lane one and drew even with him with 10 meters to go. Just before the finish line, Richard's foot landed on the inside curb as he exchanged elbows with #7. He dove at the line and landed on his face.

The medics helped Richard and #7—who turned out to be his friend, Joe Hall—to the medical tent and then to the Competitor's Room. Together, Richard and Joe watched the finish of their race on tape delay. They laughed at the elbowing incident. But they still didn't know who finished seventh and made it, and who finished eighth and would be watching.

Forty minutes later the results were posted. Cook won the heat in 8:29.67. Johnny was fourth in 8:30.54—his second personal best of the meet. Richard and Joe were listed as running the same time 8:37.21—a personal best for both—but Richard was listed as seventh and Joe as eighth. Joe protested his placement, and, after much reviewing of the photo finish, was granted a spot in the final on Friday.

To celebrate, Richard and Joe bought each other a round on Bourbon Street and toasted to their success in sneaking into what was now the Elite 15.

The Final

On Friday, Richard woke up around 9 a.m. Johnny was gone. They'd been in New Orleans, living in the same hotel room for six days, and Richard had spoken about ten words to Johnny since they left Arboretum. This wasn't the way he wanted to end it—with the silent treatment from his hero. But he'd made a commitment to himself, and Richard was never one to back down on a commitment.

He wondered, as he sat alone at breakfast, if he had done something to piss Johnny off. He couldn't think of anything. He decided it was just Johnny acting weird during the most important and stressful meet of his life.

The Olympic Trials are a real make-it or break-it meet for many people. And at the age of 26, Johnny was at one of those crossroads in life. If he did well, he could justify committing another four years of his life to working part-time for shit pay, while making the rest of his puny income in the unpredictable field of road racing.

At the next trials, Johnny would be 30. Was he willing to hold off on "growing up" and joining the real world for another four years? Most who don't make the Olympic team are not. Not at the age of 26, anyway. That's why making it was so important to Johnny.

Richard could see where Johnny was coming from. He understood Johnny's anti-social behavior and didn't take it personally.

Joe Hall came over to Richard's table and sat down. They talked over breakfast about some of the results from the meet and even talked a little about race strategy.

After breakfast, the two took a leisurely walk to the Quarter and hung out in a few bookstores. They walked back to the hotel around noon, ate lunch, and then went back to Joe's room and hung out.

"Hey, Richard," Joe said. "I was talking to some of the sprinters on your team after the SEC meet. They said that you don't sleep the night before you race. And that you pace the floor and think about killing the guys in the race. Is that true?"

"Well, sprinters have a way of embellishing things," Richard said, a little embarrassed. "But it's true to some degree. I don't sleep well the night before races. I get about six hours the night before most races, which isn't bad. But for meets like the NCAAs and SECs—especially the SECs—I get between one and three."

"Holy shit! How do you race the next day?"

"I don't know. I just do."

"How many hours did you sleep before you won the SEC Indoor 3K?"

"Maybe two?"

"Son of a bitch," Joe said. "Did you want to kill me before the race?"

"Hell, no, Joe. I just wanted to win real bad. I don't want to kill anyone. . . except myself on occasion." There was an awkward silence. Joe didn't know how to respond to the strange statement. Richard realized this and tried to smooth things over.

"And of course those Arkansas bastards," he added. Joe chuckled and the awkward moment was forgotten.

"I've looked in your eyes before a race," Joe said. "You may not want to kill people, but you're out for blood, man. I've seen it. It's intimidating. . . You know, you're lucky. Sometimes I have so much trouble getting motivated to race. I wish I had that kind of intensity at racetime."

"No you don't, Joe. It's more of a curse than anything. Believe me," Richard said, choosing to end it with that comment, rather than describe one of the many nights he seemed headed for a nervous breakdown.

Richard went back to his room around 3 p.m. and took a nap. It was going to be a long night and he wanted to be awake and aware for the whole thing.

He woke at 4:30 and threw his uniform and spikes into the bag. His racing shirt—an old, cut-up, khaki green T-shirt he got for 99 cents at an Army-Navy store in Arboretum—reeked because it hadn't been washed since his arrival in New Orleans. Richard was running better than he had all season and superstition had caught up with him. He didn't want to wash the "lucky sweat" off the uniform that had gotten him into the Olympic Trials final. As he put the uniform in the bag he realized that the lucky sweat was a little more than he had bargained for.

Richard went downstairs to grab a roll on his way out. As he went out to wait for the bus he saw Joe Hall. The two sat together on the bus over to the track. Richard had liked Joe before the Olympic Trials week. But it was in a distant way. Since they competed for different schools in the same event, they never got to know each other except as friendly rivals. But spending time together in New Orleans, they had developed a bond. They had even adopted a kind of team mentality by agreeing to work together in the early part of the final.

With Johnny off in his own world of mental torture, Joe had unknowingly helped Richard take his mind off the mission. Richard was much more relaxed about finishing the mission, thanks to Joe.

"You nervous?" Joe asked Richard on the bus ride over to the track. "You don't look it."

"Nah, I ain't nervous. I reached my goal. I got here."

"I feel the same way," Joe smiled. "I was nervous before the first two rounds. But now that I'm in the final I've got nothing to lose. I've already made it further than I thought I would."

"I haven't had more than a few pre-race jitters in a while," Richard said.

"What about the conference meet a few weeks ago?" Joe said. "I thought you slept only a few hours during that meet."

"I did," Richard said. "But it wasn't because I was nervous about winning. That's what used to keep me up. At SECs that first night, I stayed awake because I felt like staying awake. Not because I was nervous."

"You're full of shit," Joe said.

"No, I'm dead serious," Richard responded. "A few weeks before SECs I made peace with myself. I just decided that enough was enough. I made a decision that I wasn't going to lose sleep over winning and losing anymore. I was just going to give my best effort, and whatever happened, I'd live with the results. I figured that I might as well enjoy my last few track meets and remember them fondly, instead of through the dark glasses that I remember every other track meet that was important in my life."

"Wow!" Joe exclaimed. "So you're saying this is it? Retirement after tonight?"

"Yep."

"Are you sure you're ready to end it all tonight?"

"I've given that subject a lot of thought, Joe. And I think tonight is a very good night to end it all," Richard said, looking evenly at Joe.

"Well, I hope it ends the way you've planned," said Joe.

"I'm sure it will," Richard said, unsmiling.

When the two got to the track, they checked in and hung out at the warm-up area until 6 p.m. On their warm-up Richard and Joe discussed strategy for the first three laps of the race. Richard said he wanted to stay near the leaders. "We're here. We might as well put ourselves in a position to win the thing," he said. Joe liked the idea, but worried that if the pace was too fast at the start, they would drop like flies after the mile mark.

"Let's just say 'Fuck it!'" Richard said. "Let's find Mike Cook and stick to him as long as we can. He knows what he's doing. I have a feeling, the longer we stay with him, the closer we'll be to maybe stealing a spot on The Team."

Joe liked the sound of "The Team" and agreed.

Richard got a warm feeling as he entered the stadium. Looking out into the packed stands, he was full of emotion. He could feel a lump begin to grow in his throat and tears begin to well up in his eyes. He had been able to hold it off for weeks. But here in New Orleans, in the biggest race of his life, it had finally hit him that this would be the last race of his life—no matter the outcome.

All of this emotion was not good, he told himself while doing his pre-race strides. Emotion in a distance race lasts for a quarter-mile and tends to drain an athlete in the latter stages of the race. So he wiped away his tears, and in doing so, wiped away the emotion. He stepped to the line and awaited the inevitable.

While staring at the ground, waiting for the starter's commands, Richard heard someone in the stands shout, "Let's go, Johnny and Dick. . . Kick some ass!"

Richard looked up for a moment and met eyes with Hargrove in the stands. Richard smiled and gave him the thumbs up sign. He looked over at Johnny, who was staring straight ahead and didn't acknowledge Hargrove's presence. Richard felt guilty for looking up at Hargrove, instead of concentrating on the task at hand. He stared back at the ground and awaited the call to the line.

When the gun went off, he looked to his right and saw Joe struggling immediately. He looked ahead and saw the reason for the struggle. The lead pack had taken to sprinting the first 100 meters. The group was lead by Mike Cook, who was followed closely by Johnny.

Before Richard knew what hit him, he was in dead last, just behind his buddy Joe Hall. Richard hung in the back for the first lap, then pulled up beside Joe, motioning him to move up.

The pace hadn't slowed much by the time the racers hit the first water jump, but Richard and Joe moved up slowly through the pack anyway. By the time they hit the water jump on the second lap, they were nestled in behind Cook. Johnny had settled into the middle of the pack and looked tired when Richard passed him. Neither of them had ever run a steeplechase at this pace.

Richard felt great both mentally and physically. He wasn't intimidated at all. The longer the race went on, the more Richard believed that he truly could make The Team.

After the third water jump, Richard looked over at Joe and saw that the torturous pace was wearing him out. They went over a few hurdles before Richard looked over again. Joe had faded and was no longer in sight.

Coming into the fourth water jump, Richard was beginning to feel the effects of it all—the pace and the two rounds of steeples just to make it to this race, not to mention all of the racing he'd done in the previous three weeks. He was hoping the others were getting tired too and would slow down. It didn't happen, though.

With three laps remaining, Mike Cook picked up the pace, as if the first $4^1/2$ laps were a jog. A group of runners went with Cook. Among them was Johnny, who looked only slightly worse than he did on the second lap.

In a matter of seconds, Richard went from second place to seventh. And he was powerless to do anything about it. There would be no last lap heroics by Richard Dubin in this race, and he knew it.

With the race essentially over for Richard, he had two choices. He could put his head down and fight as hard as he could to hold his position, which was highly unlikely, anyway. Or he could half-ass it and watch the end of the race as he jogged it in. He wanted to give everything he had, but his body had nothing left to give. And since he was no longer fighting for a spot on The Team, he couldn't help but glance occasionally towards the lead pack which was increasing its lead on him at an alarming rate.

Richard was approaching his sixth water jump and he heard

a bell ring. He looked up for a brief moment to see that the leaders were crossing the finish line and had one lap to go. Only five remained, and Cook and Johnny were two of them. Richard looked ahead at his water jump and stepped over it surprisingly well considering how tired he was. "Only one more of those to go," he told himself.

After Richard cleared the next hurdle, he looked again at the leaders and saw that they'd picked up the pace yet again. Cook was still the leader, but the pack had been pared to four. Johnny was still in there, but he was hanging on like a man being dragged by a horse. He had nothing left. All he had to do was beat one guy, though. The question at that point was: Did he have enough left to do it?

Richard crossed the finish line, cleared the hurdle just beyond it and then looked to the other end of the track where the leaders were approaching the water jump for the last time. Cook sped up, stepped on the barrier, pushed off and barely got one foot wet. It was picture-perfect.

The three right behind Cook were not nearly as smooth. The guys in second and third stepped on the barrier together. Both landed ankle deep in the water. An exhausted Johnny in desperation attacked the water jump and hurdled it, landing shin deep in the water. He stumbled out of the water pit—his aggressiveness costing him precious meters. With 120 meters to go, Johnny had his head down and looked as if he'd given up.

Richard, now on the backstretch of his last lap, looked ahead toward the next hurdle he had to clear with the assumption that Johnny's Trials had ended with that water jump. But legends like Johnny don't go down with 120 meters to go. They go down to the wire.

Richard cleared that hurdle and looked over to see Johnny—head still down in an all-out sprint. He hurdled the final barrier in stride and continued his sprint. Johnny was making up ground on the three in front of him with every step he took. But with 60 meters left he still had 10 meters to make up. Was there enough track to catch someone?

Richard looked ahead just in time to jump over the next hurdle. Another second of leader-watching and he would have crashed into the 75-lb. barrier. He looked over as he was about to enter the curve toward his last water jump. He saw Johnny making up even more ground.

Forty meters left: Johnny was seven meters back. Richard, who entered the curve, was losing sight of the finishers. Thirty meters left: Johnny was five meters back. Twenty meters left: three meters back. Ten meters left: one meter back. Finish line: Richard looked ahead stutter-stepped over the barrier and landed knee-deep in the water pit.

With one runner 20 yards ahead and two about the same distance behind, Richard gave a half-hearted effort at a sprint in the final home stretch. As he ran toward the finish line, he heard the sympathy clap from the crowd that said, "Well, you didn't make The Team, but you gave a good effort anyway, and we appreciate it."

What a way to end a career, he thought. With the sympathy clap.

Richard crossed the finish line and walked toward the outside lanes. He lay down on the track, partly out of exhaustion, and partly because he wanted to soak in a few more moments of this magical experience before they escorted him off forever.

From the ground he looked at the applauding fans in the packed stadium, and then up at the stars, which shone brightly on the clear night—a rarity in New Orleans. It was a beautiful view of the world. But after a few minutes, two trainers came and lifted him off the ground, shoved a cup of water in his hand and escorted him out of the stadium to the recovery area.

As they led him away from the finish chute, Richard looked over his shoulder to get one last picture in his head. And then it was gone.

While lying on a table in the recovery area, he thought little about his race. He finished in 12th place with a time of 8:58.38—subpar at best—but he didn't care. He accomplished what he set out to do. Now he just wanted to drink a few beers with his friends and end his mission the way he'd planned.

"How'd you feel?" came a voice. It was Joe.

"Good for the first half. Shitty for the second half," Richard said as he sat up. "How 'bout you?"

"Good for the first lap. Shitty for every other one," he said. "I finished 14th in about 9:05."

"Hey, at least you didn't finish last," Richard said.

"I'll drink to that tonight," Joe said.

"Joe, do you know if Johnny made the team?"

"I think he finished fourth."

"Fourth! Are you sure?" Richard asked.

"That's just what I heard," Joe said cautiously. "I haven't seen the official results. I heard the top four guys ran really fast."

"No shit!"

Richard and Joe watched the tape of the race in the recovery area. The race was every bit as exciting as Richard remembered. He was proud to be a part of it, despite his last few laps. With the camera at the finish line, he still couldn't tell for sure if Johnny was third or fourth. But he had a sneaking suspicion that Joe was right. When the results came out, Richard read them and nearly wept:

1. Mike Cook 8:16.69
2. David Abetemarco 8:16.87
3. Stan Hurst...................................... 8:16.91
4. Johnny Reilly 8:16.92

Johnny had run his third personal best of the meet, but that was no consolation. He was still fourth—by 1/100 of a second.

After Richard read the results, he went on an all-out search for Johnny. He wanted to see him, to tell him something, anything that would make him feel like he accomplished something by "almost making The Team." But it was to no avail. He was gone. The top four finishers were taken to the interview room, then the drug testing room, and were then released.

Richard left Joe and caught the bus back to the hotel. He ran upstairs, but Johnny had already come and gone. He threw his stuff down in frustration and sat on his bed. He wanted to rush out the door. But he had business to attend to first.

Richard had promised himself that on his final night he would not write a suicide note. He feared that such a note might bring out strong emotions that would make him reconsider the mission. But he did want to leave something for Johnny.

Richard's hero was hurting, and there was no way to say what he wanted to say through speech. So he violated his rule and wrote Johnny a letter:

Johnny Boy,

By the time you read this note, I should already be gone. I've given a lot of thought to my life in its current state, and I've decided it is unacceptable.

As you well know, I've always put a lot of pressure on myself to attain certain goals. But the limited success I've achieved has not justified the mental and physical torture I've been putting myself through over the past five years.

I've tried to take the easy-going approach to running that you have. But I just can't take setbacks in stride, nor fully enjoy victory like you. I've tried, and it just doesn't work for me. Because of that, I've decided that changes need to be made. And I've made them.

Attached to this note is my ring from our SEC Cross Country Championship five years ago. It means more to me than any of my possessions. This ring not only represents what I still consider to be my finest moment as an athlete, it represents our friendship and a bond by which we will always be tied.

I want you to know how proud I am of your effort tonight. Even though you finished fourth, you've never looked finer than you did in that last 100 meters of the race. You're truly an inspiration to anyone who knows the meaning of the word "effort."

In that light, I hope you don't decide to make this latest effort your last. You're a great warrior and our sport would suffer in your absence. But, then again, you must do what you feel is best for you. I must do the same.

Your Friend,
Dick

When he finished writing, he folded up the note and put it and the ring on Johnny's bed. He hopped in the shower, threw on some clothes, and went out in search of his hero.

ZERO

Last Night on Earth

Richard wandered through the streets of the French Quarter looking for Johnny. Although he couldn't catch up with Johnny, he figured Hargrove had. And if Hargrove was with him, they had to be drinking. He stopped in numerous bars, looked around, recognized no one, and continued on his quest.

After about 30 minutes of searching bars in the Quarter, Richard walked into one and found Johnny, Hargrove, and a bunch of other people he didn't recognize at a table drinking beer. He was relieved.

The other people adjusted their chairs when they realized that Richard intended to sit down next to Hargrove and across from Johnny.

"What's up?" Johnny said. He had a look in his eye Richard had never seen before. He couldn't tell if it was a look of contentment and peace or utter hopelessness. Either way, it worried Richard because he doubted if Johnny ever felt any of those emotions. Johnny was a fighter. He was never content unless he won, and he was never hopeless.

"How do you feel now?" Richard asked cautiously.

"I feel all right. I'm a little sore, but I'll get over it."

"Same here," said Richard, who had downed some aspirin to relieve the cramps in his legs that were inevitable after three steeplechases in five days. "Are you going over to Europe to race?"

"I'm not sure. I'm really not sure what I'm going to do now."

"Well, you just got three PR's in one week. Maybe you should go to Disney World."

The joke brought a brief smile to Johnny's face. But it quickly faded back to the melancholy look he'd had before.

What's wrong with you? Richard wanted to ask. When your career was in the toilet you always had a smile on your face. Now that you've just resurrected it, you're sad? He said nothing, though, and just stared.

"I suppose I'm happy with my performance," Johnny said, leaning forward so he could talk without everyone else hearing. "But I just can't help thinking that I ran my best—the best I'm ever gonna run. I'll probably never run faster than I did tonight. And it still wasn't good enough to make The Team. My window of opportunity was open and I was one hundredth of a second slow."

Richard heard a frustration in Johnny's voice that he knew very well. But he'd never heard it from Johnny before. Richard wondered: Did he feel this way all along? Or did all this come upon him when he saw the photo finish which showed him to be the odd man out?

"Dude, I'm going to take a walk," Johnny said.

Richard wanted to join him. He wanted to say more, but he couldn't find the right words to say. He also could tell that Johnny wanted to be by himself and sort out his feelings. He understood where Johnny was coming from and regrettably watched him walk away.

He felt sorry for him, but he couldn't let Johnny's sadness ruin his last evening on Earth. He went to the bar, bought two beers, sat down next to Hargrove and said, "Let's drink."

Hargrove was more than happy to oblige. The two drank for hours. Later in the evening, Joe caught up with them and they drank some more. At 3 a.m. Richard walked Hargrove back to his hotel in the Quarter.

Hanging out with Hargrove had put a buzz on Richard, but he was not so far gone that he couldn't function. He didn't want his last moments on Earth to be spent in a drunken stupor. At the same time, he wasn't going to get all emotional about it. He didn't want his last moments to be sad moments, like saying good-bye to the trees and buildings or something corny like that. And if he started saying "Good-bye" to people in an overly emotional way, somebody might start to suspect something and attempt to talk him out of his mission.

Richard also feared that if he got too emotional about his last hours he might do something stupid like start looking at pictures of his family. All this sadness might convince him to abort the mission, which he couldn't do. He'd made a commitment to himself and he couldn't respect himself if he broke that commitment.

Emotion had almost overcome him on a few occasions in the weeks since his decision. Each time he had been able to brush it aside. But each time the emotions came stronger, and it became harder to ignore them. He was able to calm himself down, though, by reminding himself of the mission and how it must be completed. "Better to just be emotionless," he told himself, "and enjoy your remaining hour."

It was 3:20 a.m. when Richard got back to his room. The light and fan were on in the bathroom with the door closed. Richard had had more than a few beers and needed badly to empty his bladder.

"Hurry up, Johnny, I'm seeing yellow," Richard said quietly.

He looked over at Johnny's bed and got a chill. When he wrote the note, he didn't plan on being around when Johnny read it. He saw that the note and the ring hadn't been touched and was relieved. He's probably too drunk to notice, he thought, and let out a big sigh. He took the note off the bed and hid it in Johnny's bag. This way, he wouldn't find it until he unpacked when he got home.

Richard waited a few minutes and Johnny still hadn't come out of the bathroom. He was too lazy to take the elevator all the way downstairs to the lobby bathroom to take a piss. He had to go badly and he had to go now. He decided to knock.

"Hurry up, Johnny. I gotta take a leak," he said against the door. No answer. "Johnny, you all right?" he asked while knocking.

No answer. He turned the handle and the door was locked.

"Shit! Man, why'd you have to pass out with the door locked," he whined, with his head against the door.

Richard continued to knock, but there was no response from the other side of the door. He had his hand on his crotch trying to hold back the rising tide in his bladder. He couldn't make it downstairs to the lobby bathroom now, even if he wanted to. He decided in his less-than-sober state that he was going to have to bust down the door if he was to avoid wetting his pants.

He put his shoulder into the door but it didn't open. Not enough force, he thought.

The second time he stood back and came into the door with his shoulder. It budged, but still didn't open.

In desperation he took a four-step running start and launched himself into the door which flew open upon contact.

Richard couldn't control his momentum when the door came open. He slipped on the wet bathroom floor as he came in. As he was falling he could see Johnny in his peripheral vision, passed out in the tub.

Richard fell hard and banged his head on the tile floor. He lay there stunned for a moment and laughed at himself for being so clumsy. He thought Johnny must have taken a shower and drip-dried on the floor to make the tile so slippery. He felt the back of his head instinctively to make sure his brains hadn't fallen out: the old "examine the hand to make sure the head's all right" trick. His hand came back red.

"Holy shit. I must have fallen hard," he said in response to the blood on his hand.

He lifted his head and looked toward the tub. He saw his gun laying on the floor beside the tub. His eyes traveled further north and he saw Johnny motionless, with his head leaning over the side of the tub.

Richard saw the pool of red under Johnny's head. The pool now covered much of the bathroom floor. He saw a large red stain splattered against the back wall of the tub and smaller splatter stains on the tile of the other tub walls.

Richard gasped in shock. Johnny had shot himself through the mouth with the gun that was supposed to end Richard's life. When everything hit home to Richard, he involuntarily added his own urine to the pool of his friend's blood, in which he was now covered.

Moving On

Richard had always bragged that he could pack up his entire life into his car and be gone in less than an hour, if he ever needed to get out of town in a hurry.

He was surprised though when he got back to the house Monday at about 3 in the afternoon; his boasting had been accurate. In 45 minutes the car was practically full with only a few more items to collect.

Phil came home from school and saw that Richard was packing his car to leave. Phil was fully aware of everything that had happened, as it was all over the newspaper by then. He knew that Richard had been through the wringer, losing a close friend and being questioned by the police for hours. He knew that he'd been kept in a jail cell for more than two days before be-

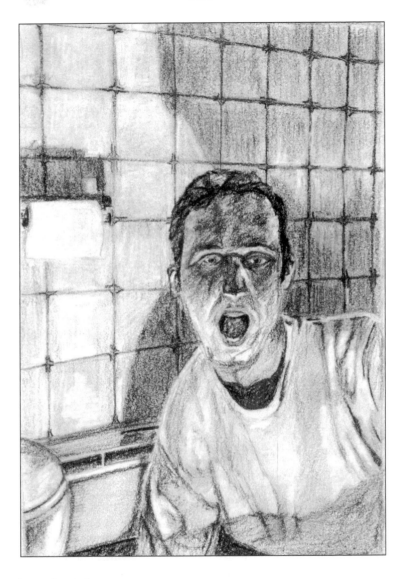

ing released.

According to the newspapers, Richard confessed to buying the handgun to use in his own suicide attempt. There were three bullets left in the gun's chamber with which he could have completed his mission, but he lost his will to die while lying in the blood of his friend and hero.

He told police that finding Johnny in that condition changed his perspective on life and death. He wouldn't elaborate on his new perspective, except to say, "Suicide is a lot more horrible than I ever imagined."

Knowing all this, Phil felt awkward about saying anything to him.

4 p.m. Now only Richard's bed, dresser, and desk remained in his room. Those items were given to him by past roommates. In Arboretum tradition, he asked Phil to give them to whoever needed them, and to put any of the unwanted items by the dumpster where they were sure to find a loving home.

Phil understood the drill and knew of people, including himself, who could use the items left behind.

Richard checked over the apartment once more to make sure he hadn't missed anything he needed. He didn't want to have to go through the trouble of asking Phil to send him anything through the mail. Not that Phil wouldn't have. Richard just wanted to make a clean break from the town without leaving any trace that he'd been there.

He went out to shut the hatchback to his car, which he'd parked about three feet from the front door on the grass, when he heard the phone ring. Phil picked it up on the second ring. Richard could hear him whispering into the phone. He wanted to make a clean getaway and he looked at Phil, praying the call wasn't for him. He prayed even harder that it wasn't Susan. His prayers went unanswered.

Phil looked at Richard as he stood in the doorway and mouthed her name so she couldn't hear. Richard looked down and began to feel his throat and eyes swell.

"I can't. I gotta go," he said weakly.

Phil, who held the phone at his hip, left the receiver uncovered so she could hear every word Richard said. Phil watched as Richard tried to hold himself together. Phil could hear a faint sound of crying from the receiver.

Getting it from both ends, Phil's throat began to tighten as well. "Where are you going?" Phil asked.

"I'm not sure," Richard said, still looking at the ground trying to collect himself. Why can't you hold it together in these situations, he thought to himself. "I think I might move up to North Carolina. I heard the mountains in the western part of the state are beautiful." he said, leaning against the door frame and staring off into the trees beside the house.

"You want me to say anything to Susan?" Phil asked.

"Yeah," he paused a few seconds to collect himself and looked at Phil. "A friend once told me that I was a good person and I should allow myself to have a good life. He said I deserved it. Tell her. . ."

He stopped for a moment. He was falling apart again. He looked out at the trees again through moist eyes and took a calming breath to collect himself.

"Tell her I said she deserves it, too," he said and turned towards his car.

Phil nodded gravely and spoke into the receiver. Richard could hear a soft tearful response on the other end.

"Hey," Phil called solemnly. Richard paused with the handle to the car door in his hand and looked at Phil. "If you ever get lonely up in the mountains don't be afraid to come down and see us some day."

Looking at the ground, Richard paused to think about it. He knew he could never come back to Arboretum. Too many ghosts. But standing in front of Phil (and Susan) was not the time to say "never."

He looked at Phil, took one more deep breath to settle his quaking chest, and said in a voice strong enough to be heard over the phone line, "Some day."

He got in his car and drove off, closing a chapter in his life that he could only measure in degrees of pain.